THE OTHER SIDE
OF THE
MEDICAL COIN

THE OTHER SIDE
OF THE
MEDICAL COIN

DESMOND S.

Library of Congress Control Number: 2011960133
ISBN: Hardcover   978-1-4653-9222-0
                  Softcover   978-1-4653-9221-3
                  Ebook   978-1-4653-9223-7

This book was printed in the United States of America.

To order additional copies of this book, contact:
Xlibris Corporation
1-888-795-4274
www.Xlibris.com
Orders@Xlibris.com
89606

CONTENTS

To all the nurses and patients, the World over

My wife, Martha Ann,

My daughter, Amanda Marie

And all of my peers.

I would like to pay my homage to the military for their sacrifice and dedication in keeping America safe. (From a vet)

PREFACE

After pondering for years, often daily and with the encouragement of my peers, I have finally decided to write this book on medical issues, nursing errors, doctors' misdiagnoses, and patient abuses.

The aim of this presentation is not to condemn nurses or doctors but more to inform them and the public that these errors are real and have already occurred. If they are aware that it is possible for these mistakes to recur, then it is my wish and hope that they will take all the necessary precautions to prevent them.

It is my utmost desire to inform patients of the risks associated with hospitalization and of what to look for as nurses and doctors treat and attend to them. It is not my intention for my readers to interpret this information as in any way condescending, and for all it's worth, they should adhere to the advice of the medical team after weighing the preponderance of all options.

Please be aware that no one is all perfect, but an accountant can correct his numbers; sometimes it is difficult, highly improbable, or even impossible to correct medical errors.

My personal religious beliefs are related to my culture, and in no way am I trying to convert anyone to my religion.

A SHORT AUTOBIOGRAPHY

I was born in British Guiana, now a republic with the name changed to Guyana. I grew up with my grandmother, grandfather, stepaunts, and stepuncles from the tender age of six months old. My adoption materialized from the fact that four serious operations were performed on me, my mom was nineteen years old, and everyone thought it best for me to be taken care of by my more experienced grandparents.

I was literally spoiled rotten by my grandfather and his children. I got everything I wanted but did not necessarily need. My aunt even sewed and knitted my clothes, and I was taken for a walk every day. My grandfather had rice land and owned a little shop that sold bread, cakes, soft drinks, and some haberdashery. The town was named New Amsterdam, with a relative population of approximately seven thousand people. The population was exclusively of African and East Indian decent. It was an insult and almost considered a crime to refer to people by the color of their skin. There were about five families in New Amsterdam that were consistent with my color, and none were my family or friends.

In primary school, there were only two other boys with the same color as I, so I stood out among my peers. This unfortunate distinction motivated me to perform at my highest potential, for I was easily recognized in a group, be it good or bad. This distinction was also responsible for my meticulous enthusiasm. This craving for perfection served me well in later life but also became an obsession. I still hate to be wrong or ignorant of so many things; however, I am very aware of my limits. If I decide to accept a challenge, I will dedicate myself to that feat, or I would never attempt it.

At the age of eleven and up, I started high school. I did my best to attain academic excellence and, at the same time, to maintain a high degree of physical fitness. I joined judo and boxing clubs and always maintained my presence in the defensive arts. I never retreated, regardless of the opponents' size or age, although it was not always in my best interest. The big guys, I observed, relied on their size and voice, which apparently emphasized their dominance; nevertheless, I developed the courage to stand up and fight for my rights and sometimes my life. This ultimately prevented many from even thinking about tangling with me—and my defense. For those who are bullied, please remember that these bullies have probably never been hit physically, but if you are being punched, the only alternative is to punch back. Surprisingly, this may end the encounter and even prevent others from attempting to bully you.

At the time I attended school, corporal punishment was the rule of the era. In primary school, lashes with a "wild cane" of about three to four feet in length were the usual punishment for tardiness and errors in subjects of math, English, history, and even religion. I attended a Roman Catholic school, which undoubtedly had a higher standard of education than the other schools. There was one significant punishment on Mondays for those with more than four errors in spelling from dictation. This exercise was done by the teacher reading a passage from a book, and pupils had to write with correct spelling what she dictated. I have always stated my disgust with this form of punishment. The most I was disciplined for was tardiness. Talking in class, disrupting the class, cursing, and insubordination were always dealt with severely.

I excelled in mathematics, the sciences, literature, and Latin. I also took scripture as a subject and studied the Gospels of Matthew, Mark, John, and the Acts of the Apostles. I was also an altar boy in the Roman Catholic Church for several years, and may I say, no priest ever looked at me indifferently.

After graduating from school, I taught at different schools as an assistant teacher, was the manager of three huge hardware warehouses, a customs officer, and a payroll clerk called a paymaster. I also worked as an insurance underwriter for three companies and, finally, was a soldier for many years in different armies. Finally, I became an ear, nose, and throat specialist and performed a very exclusive technical test called electronystagmography—a test that compares the balance organs in both ears, may suggest that there is something wrong with the cranial eight nerve and because cold and warm water is used in the ear to induce nystagmus, information gathered from the comparison of the direction of the nystagmus is used to investigate the vestibular cochlea labyrinth. I will go into further explanation to show how this test is used because the dictionary gives a definition of electronystamography as that pertaining to the eyes. This information is written mainly for nurses and doctors as it deals intensely with anatomy and physiology, which takes years to grasp, understand and remember. If you are not medically oriented, this explanation is not meant for you. There are numerous data that can be gathered from the eyes. The eyes can almost determine over a hundred pieces of information. There are three parts in the ear. The outer ear, the middle ear, and the inner ear. The inner ear is connected to the outer ear by the tympanic membrane of which a small bony structure called the malleus is attached and which is cemented and joined to the incus, which is joined to the stapes and to the inner ear labyrinth. The inner ear consists of two parts, the bony labyrinth and the membranous labyrinth. There are three parts to the bony labyrinth, the vestibule, cochlea and the semicircular canals. The membranous labyrinth consists of the utricle and saccule inside the vestibule, the cochlear duct is inside the cochlea and the membranous semicircular canals are inside the bony ones.

The membranous utricle and saccule are suspended within the vestibule. They are separated from the bony walls of the vestibule by fluid (perilymph), and both utricle and saccule contains a fluid called endolymph. Located within the utricle (and also within the saccule) lies a small structure called the macula. It consists mainly of hair cells and a gelatinous membrane that contains otoliths (tiny 'stones'—that is, small particles of calcium carbonate). A few delicate hairs protrude from the hair cells and are embedded in the gelatinous membrane.

Receptors for the vestibular branch of the eight cranial nerve contact the hair cells of the macula located in the utricle. Changing position of the head to induce nystagmus, and using cold and then warm water in the head, causes a change in the amount of pressure on the gelatinous membrane and causes the otoliths to pull on the hair cells. This stimulates the adjacent receptors of the vestibular nerve. Its fibers conduct impulses to the brain which produce a sense of the position of the head and also a sensation of a change in the pull of gravity.

In addition, stimulation of the macula in the utricle evokes righting reflexes, muscular responses to restore the body and its parts to their normal position when they have been displaced. Impulses from proprioceptors and from the eyes also activate righting reflexes. Interruption of the vestibular or visual or proprioceptive impulses that initiate these reflexes may cause disturbances of equilibrium, nausea, vomiting and other symptoms.

That is the connection between the eyes and the ears. Police uses the eyes for various drug and alcohol tests. Physicians test the eyes of boxers after they are knocked down and also after the fight.

The test of electronystamography consist of electrodes placed at specific places around the eyes, and the patient is asked to look right and left a number of times, usually as a base line but sometimes unusual patterns are observed. The patient is placed down and up in a rapid movement while recording eye movement. Last but not least, cold water and then warm water is poured into the ear for two minutes each, each ear, and this produces rapid nystagmus. The form, consistency, height, and duration is determined and simple mathematical calculations are performed. So the definition in the Merriam-Webster dictionary, although being correct, does not give the relationship between the ear and the eye.

After three years as an ear, nose, and throat specialist and after completing several college courses, I was offered a nineteen thousand—dollar bonus to complete a licensed vocational nurse (LVN) course—which lasted two years—and I couldn't let that offer pass. I graduated from this grueling course, and I use that term loosely because it not only prepared me as an LVN but maintained my fitness for combat duty. I was sent to Germany, which in part halted my educational progress toward becoming a registered nurse, but I continued to study; and as soon as I returned to the United States, I became a registered nurse. I had already taken ACLS (advanced cardiac life support) and was an ACLS instructor. I have taught and tested nurses, physicians and emergency medical technicians in helping to diagnose, treat with chest compressions and drugs in emergencies. Every nurse and doctor should take and pass ACLS.

By this time, I suffered from chest pain while running during physical training, and I observed multiple changes on my electrocardiogram. I saw several doctors, including a PA (physician's assistant), on sick call. They almost had me believing that there was nothing wrong and that the pain was perceived erroneously in my head. Finally, after I knew it was not fictitious, I requested that my commander release me; I had only months to fulfill my contract. He did. Ironically, however, I did prove, to my detriment, that these doctors who I saw were incorrect, especially that PA. A year after I left the army, I had a four-vessel heart bypass surgery performed on me emergently.

As a registered nurse, I continued to work in the ICU (intensive care unit) and the ER (emergency room). My ideal patients were trauma patients. The hospital I worked at in California was about one mile away from the prison. And every night, be it prisoners or civilians, there were always excitement in the ER and subsequently the ICU—with patients recovering from multiple stab wounds, gunshot wounds and attempted suicide, illicit drug overdosed patients. As morbid as it sounds, this presented a challenge for excellence in care and interventions.

Soon after I was employed at this hospital, I was notified by the Union that if I did not subscribe to Union dues, they would recommend that I be fired. I felt distraught because I thought that America was the "land of the free and brave" and a democracy. I was never threatened with my livelihood before, and I was not only astounded but angry that so few were dictating the rules of so many. I did not belong to any political party, but that was my honest view. I thought that I should be hired, promoted, or even fired by my performance. Fortunately, I did not have to endure this injustice too long because my wife, who is also an ICU nurse, did not entertain the small earth tremors/earthquakes, so we moved to another state.

At my next assignment, I started in a surgical intensive care unit (SICU). As an LVN, I was trained to care for medical intensive care unit (MICU) patients, and in Germany, I mainly took care of cardiac patients along with some medical and post-op patients. This was a challenge for me because I remembered that surgical nurses always had that special confidence and knowledge of proficiency that I admired. I not only learned the art of setting up Swan-Ganz and arterial catheters, but I was able to compute and determine cardiac output, pulmonary arterial pressures, and wedges and could actually say what the blood pressure was at any one time. I learned how to perform arterial punctures for blood gases with great precision. Inserting Foleys, rectal tubes and bags became second nature.

However, with all the technology of a Swan-Ganz, there is no literature that supports a Swan-Ganz has been used to prevent morbidity. The entire cardiac output and oxycalculation (oxygen calculation called oxycals) from a Swan-Ganz numbers are fantastic and may help in severe sepsis/shock, but the best outcomes are from what the doctors do with this information. I also worked with continuous dialysis machines, from setting them up to effective meticulous monitoring. I have taken care of postoperative open heart valve and heart vessel bypass patients. I have seen the effects of vasodilators, hypotensive drugs, and beta-blockers; treated patients with tachycardia through drugs and by electrical cardioversion and performed multiple heart compressions, an integral part of basic cardiac life support (BCLS), and shocked patients who are in ventricular fibrillation.

My knowledge and experience allowed me to perform conscious sedation on patients undergoing endoscopies/colonoscopies and recovering them postoperatively. I had to do a test yearly to qualify for that assignment. I spent a little over a year in oncology, where I had the task of inserting multiple intravenous catheters on patients whose veins are fragile, almost nonexistent, from multiple sticks, effects of toxic drugs, diabetes, or kidney failure. I was also a qualified PICC insertion nurse. I soon learned to access Portacaths painlessly.

The above information is relevant to this book as it qualifies me to write this information. I did engage in a three-month stint of 'tell-a-nurse'. I officially retired in 2010, not because of my liking but because of an injury and severe medical problems. I have had ten operations performed on me. I suffer from sleep apnea, so I wear a CPAP mask during sleep. I was diagnosed with hypothyroidism and take Synthroid for that complaint; occasional congestive heart failure; arthritis to my knees, hips and fingers; congestive obstructive pulmonary disease; and severe fatigue with tiredness. There are other problems that induce pain that I tend to ignore. I have been hospitalized at least eight times. This also qualifies me to write this book from a patient's point of view.

Paradoxically, even though the nurse/doctor should be in sync with the patient, I will describe in minute detail what the patient sees of the caregivers. A point of interest is that generic drugs are only required to be 80 percent of the patient's dosage, and doctors, nurses and also patients should be very careful while switching from one to the other.

A simple calculation is that if levothyroxine is switched to Synthroid of 0.10 mg, 20 percent is added to the amount of levothyroxine, so the amount of Synthroid would be equal to 0.120 of levothyroxine. With that calculation, can you imagine how much levothyroxine equivalent you would be taking if 0.10 mg levothyroxine was raised to 0.112 mg Synthroid? The FDA requires generic drugs to be at least 80 percent of the brand name drug; I do not think in all honesty that they will produce one hundred percent in the generic drug. Pharmacists describe generic drugs as those that work in place of brand name drugs; and some generic drugs do.

MY PHILOSOPHY
DUM SPIRO SPERO

The above expression is figuratively translated as "while there is life, there is hope." I hold firm to this phrase as I have seen evidence that when all efforts are exhausted, there is always that very slim chance of recovery. That is taking all into account, sometimes it's best to end the suffering by letting go. I know that I am not God, and I am sure that you know that too; but paradoxically, the only persons who do not know that are brain surgeons.

Please bear with me for I promise you that the following chapters will surely amaze you after reading, but almost everyone, if not all, have established ideas, beliefs, and dreams that probably lead to abstract epics.

Sometimes this philosophy can be cultured by family and their customs, friends, environment, education, or even fantasy. We occasionally develop and entertain visions that ultimately turn into staunch beliefs. For instance, I am a Roman Catholic because I was "born" into the church. I was baptized, had my first Holy Communion, was confirmed, and was even an altar boy for many years. This has in no way made me more holy than anyone else, but my roots had been established and my worship of God and my belief in angels are strongly associated with the Roman Catholic Church. I can safely attribute this devotion to friends, family, and environment.

I am very aware of harsh decisions made by the pope and the church, especially against the Jews during World War II, almost taking Hitler's side on his mass eradication in the Holocaust. Every era has its follies and tribulations: the Vikings, Hannibal, Alexander, Stalin, Lenin—and more recently, Mao Tse-Tung, Castro, Assad of Syria, Chavez of Venezuela, and Idi Amin of Uganda were all brutal dictators. They are all prime examples of conquerors and dictators of the centuries past and present. There is a conservative effort presently for people of faith to coexist.

My previous qualm with the Catholic Church began as the Mass was changed from Latin to English. The priest no longer backs the congregation, but faces them behind the altar. Lay people are now qualified to give Holy Communion. I was shocked and devastated about these drastic changes initially, and I literally strayed by the wayside.

It took me years to understand that man was not made for the church, but instead, that the church was made for man and that the church will have significant changes according to evolution—but that doesn't excuse the many atrocities of the church. I have since resolved this anger that I felt for this change. In my former years, only the priest could hold the host and it should not even touch your teeth but you had to swallow it down as quickly as possible. Today, one can take the host from the priest, hold it, and chew it in one's mouth. Surely you can understand the passion I endured from this change.

I believe in God and that God is so huge and powerful that he is like unto a giant structure, like the Hoover Dam to an ant. The universe is so wide, it's impossible to fathom its length, width, and breadth. I believe that God is larger than the universe, and that explains why we don't see him; however, I also believe that supreme beings can take any form or shape. I believe in the Virgin Mary, in God the Father, God the Son, and the Holy Ghost. I believe in the saints and miracles. I also think that if I were to rake all my sins and place them into a bag, I would not be able to carry that burden. I believe that we must pray for sinners and those whom have passed.

I also now believe in UFOs. I have never disclosed this to anyone before except to my wife, for I thought that they would think I am cuckoo. But as a guard commander at an airstrip in Guyana, I once ventured outside of the guard hut for some fresh air and to admire the stars in the dark sky. I saw a light very far away in the sky, just above where I was standing, and it was slowly moving. After looking at it for a little while, this light (which I thought at first was from a jet) stopped and idled for almost fifteen minutes, then continued in the projected path. Subsequently, I read many books by Erich von Daniken, and the proposed evidence has convinced me without a doubt that there are UFOs and that—if not now, once—more civilized beings either visited, lived, or probably even mated with the people of the Earth. I believe that there is a devil with his acolytes, which brings this phenomenon to "the World of Opposites."

The World of Opposites states that if there is a man, there is a woman; if there is God, there is the devil; if there is good, there is evil; if there is hot, there is cold; if there is fire, there is water, if there is life, there is death, and so on.

I can place these phenomena on a graph of a straight line with a center X. Most people that I have interviewed think that the opposites (e.g., good and bad) begin at X, the center of the straight line, so that a little good begins at X and moves along the line increasingly to the right. A little bad starts at X and moves left along the line, increasing proportionately as it progresses. However, I think it's the opposite. The extremities of the opposites (e.g., good and bad) are at X, and they begin far away, left and right of X on the straight line. So instead of moving away from each other, they move toward each other and the extremities meet at X in the center.

My proof of this is not difficult metaphysics, for these extremities are so close to each other that they often overlap. That is why you laugh when you are too sad and you cry when you are too happy. This may also explain the actions of several preachers like Jim Jones, who murdered over one thousand persons in Guyana. Many who have crossed the barrier are extremists that initially wanted to do good for mankind but became meticulously satanic, evil, crazy, and sick. Jim Jones thought he was God and the congregation was his people. He had reached the X extremity and crossed it. That is not withholding the medical view—regardless of how crazy he was, he crossed from good to bad. I might be over reaching here because narcotics and illicit drugs were every day use. His brain may have been in a frying pan.

We, as nurses, have always said that there is more "traffic" in the emergency room when there is full moon. Well, in the hospital that I worked for in California, it must have been full moon every night, for the emergency room/trauma rooms were always full. But why should this saying be untrue? If the magnetic connection between the Earth and the moon is so great that the moon directs the tides every twelve hours and maintains the Earth in a fairly stable wobbly axis, and if our bodies contain 60 percent water, what connection do you think it has on us? Our bodies also have minerals and salts, which are also included in that great gravitational action. So I say to you that the moon does have a great influence on us—whether it's good or bad, I'll let you think about it. Without the moon as the great stabilizer, the Earth would be tumbling into the universe, and we may even fall off into space.

The sun also has a large influence on our bodies by causing skin cancer if they are exposed too long without appropriate protection. Scientists say that the moon is slowly moving away from the Earth; in this case, half an inch is an enormous catastrophe and might be, along with solar storms, responsible for our change in weather. I say so much for Al Gore's theory on Global Warming. Although I do acknowledge the fact that man is also responsible for the weather's alterations. There is also big business in initiating carbon credits and applying it the world over, but nature has a more important part in the warming. I am not asking you to believe what I write, but only to think about it. I have often thought of the mysteries of the universe, including the

Earth, sun, planets, and space. This chapter may sound like bloviating, but there must be even a little truth in what I believe. So we should now look at the real meat of this title, which is about medical errors made by both nurses and doctors.

NURSING ERRORS AND MISDIAGNOSES

If I ever state that what I write is what I heard, I'll say so; otherwise, all that I write I can safely back up because I was there. If I was ever challenged, I can prove what I write by subpoena under the freedom of information act if necessary. I'll begin with the experiences that include me as a patient. I would like to tell all caregivers who read this book to be cognizant of how a patient, lying in bed, sees the caregiver.

I had suffered a terrible right shoulder injury by trying to pull a patient, who was on a ventilator, up in bed without any help. There was no one else around, the ventilator was beeping and water was in the connecting tube. I quickly drained this condensation from the tube and realized that he was too far down in bed. You can almost drown from this condensation or acquire ventilator-assisted pneumonia if this water was transferred to your lungs.

I have been injured before doing many other things, and the pain dissipated in about three days, but this right shoulder pain got progressively worse. The pain was constant and annoying, and after a week, I finally couldn't raise my hands/arms above my shoulders. I could not hang an IV without excruciating pain. I saw several doctors about this problem, had a computerized axial tomography (CAT) scan done, and saw an orthopedic surgeon, but all treated the symptoms of pain and not the etiology.

I finally ended up in orthopedic rehab. I was given a TENS (acronym for transcutaneous electrical nerve stimulator) machine that could only run for twenty minutes at the most. It did seem to help my pain momentarily, but never completely; however, I was so glad that at least something was working. In order to save on the pads for the TENS machine, I often left them on and even left the machine attached to it. One Saturday, I awoke and immediately started the TENS treatment (the machine sends small shock waves to the injured site where the pads are placed). After about ten minutes, I began to shake and tremble tremendously. I immediately disconnected the TENS machine, but the ague continued with such ferocity that I couldn't hold a cup of coffee in my hands without spilling it.

This awful shaking and shivering continued for approximately three hours. I was taking Synthroid at that time (0.175 mg for hypothyroidism). After the shivering stopped, I got a fever of 102 degrees Fahrenheit that would not dissipate with Tylenol (625 mg every four hours). So I waited until (8:00 p.m.) that night to shower and decided to go to the hospital. I spent thirty minutes in the shower, and my wife helped me dry my feet and toes. She had been urging me to go to the hospital since this episode started, and it is important that I mention that she dried my feet after I did so, which contradicts the doctors' view that I went to the hospital with an ulcer. There were no ulcers on my ankle or lower extremities at home, both my wife and I knew that.

HYPOTHYROIDISM

The diagnosis of this disease was made by trial and error. Initially, I saw that I was losing hair on my upper legs, thighs, and ankles. All the doctors that I asked gave me a different answer; some even said that I slept on my side, and that was the reason. Some even seemed to me to make up the answers. I thought that because I had recently spent a little over a year in oncology as a nurse, I might have been affected with the effects of some toxic drug and that I may have laid a drug unconsciously on my legs while I was checking the name and dosage. I began to feel very tired, sometimes so tired that I could not get out of bed. I used a CPAP mask for sleep, so I ruled out sleep apnea. This became very distressing and irritating, and I was very baffled with this process.

I was changed from one doctor to a nurse practitioner, and I requested that she include a TSH (thyroid stimulating hormone) test in my blood's lab work. *Bingo.* The results returned with a very high TSH, which meant that I was suffering from hypothyroidism. Wouldn't you consider this as misdiagnosed? I am not sure now how many years this complaint prevailed before diagnosis, but surely, you would agree that it was misdiagnosed with all the incredible excuses I was given—from sleeping on my side to aging. I now say to doctors that if you don't know, say it as it is, "I don't know." There are a few things that I would like to review about hypothyroidism, but not going into any depth of anatomy and physiology; if I do, then I'd be straying from the main topic of errors/diagnoses.

Hypothyroidism: Some Signs and Symptoms

- Excessive hair loss
- Inability to withstand cold weather comfortably (intolerance)
- Bradycardia and/or enlarged heart
- Edema without indentation (1+, 2+, etc.)
- Vitiligo (white patches on skin, with brittle nails)
- Weakness
- Extreme tiredness with need to sleep long hours—almost unable to get out of bed
- Weight gain
- Altered night vision
- Stiff joints, like in arthritis
- Constipation

These are some of my symptoms that appeared slowly, but patients may not experience all of these and any one of these is also related to other diseases. But these were my symptoms and I couldn't relate them to hypothyroidism, but neither could the doctors I saw. And even though I didn't believe any of their answers, I was still stuck with these symptoms.

I spent about three hours in the emergency room (ER) lobby, awaiting the doctor's examination. During that time, I told the admitting nurse that I was going to take two Tylenol tabs because I felt the fever raising. He replied that he didn't hear that—meaning that he was not giving me permission to do so—but it was important for them to know so that they didn't overdose me with Tylenol. All the time in the ER, I sat in a chair with my legs down on the floor. The hospital supervisor, who I knew very well, stopped and almost kept me thinking and talking so that I almost forgot about the fever and the newly developed severe stiffness in my joints. I can't remember if I ever thanked her for the visit, but I am thanking her now. I was eventually called and led into the ER unit and placed on a bed.

The torture of starting an intravenous catheter (IV) on me began. I have very prominent veins on my hands, but after about twenty sticks, they (the nurses) were unable to insert an IV in my hands/arms. The usual way of starting an IV is to look for a blood return in the catheter before advancing the catheter into the vein. At least six nurses tried; they couldn't even get a blood stick on my finger. I knew then that my body was in, or going into, shock. The blood in my extremities was shunted from my hands, arms, and legs to my heart, lungs, kidneys, liver, and brain.

Finally, I said to the last one that if he thinks that the IV is in the vein, flush it with 10 cc (cubic centimeters) of saline, and if there was no swelling, then the IV was in. He followed my (new) instruction, and the IVs were inserted. Before this, to keep it in chronological order, the female ER doctor visited me, and the first thing she saw was that I had an ulcer on my left ankle exactly where the vein had been stripped for an open heart bypass, years ago. She asked me how long I had that ulcer. I looked down at my left ankle in awe, for there was never any ulcer there before. The ulcer was at the end of the incision.

In the meantime, another nurse was successful in drawing about 2 cc of blood from the inner aspect of my arm. I particularly asked them to include a TSH.The dosage of Synthroid that I had been taking (about three months ago) was increased from 150 mcg to 175 mcg (micrograms). My doctor had scheduled my blood test for six months instead of three, which is usually done when Synthroid is increased. Also, the increment should have been 12 mcg instead of 25. This blood was drawn before I received any fluid. I particularly mention this because later as you read on, you will find a contradiction as to when fluid was introduced.

I reiterated that I had slept with the electrodes on my skin and the TENS machine had been attached but was turned off, and they still recorded that I had slept with the TENS machine on. If they were knowledgeable on TENS machines, they would have known that they can only be set for twenty minutes at a time, the most.

I explained that the ulcer was not there when I left home, for both my wife and I had examined my feet/legs. I was rushed off to the ultrasound department where a technician was waiting. The test for blood clots or any abnormalities was completed, and I knew I did not have a clot. When I returned to the ER, the doctor told me that there were no clots and that my TSH was normal. I asked what it was, and she proudly told me that the range was from 0.33 to 5.0 and that my TSH was 0.55.

Since this incident, the values for TSH have become more stringent: they are now from 0.33 to 3.33. I intimated that for me it was very low; I've had experience with these values going under the value of 1.0, and when that occurred, I had insomnia for about three to four days (it's a horrible feeling—I can now appreciate Michael Jackson's dilemma of insomnia [RIP]). She ignored my statement, left the bedside, and ordered antibiotics—Zosyn, three doses.

I was finally taken up to a ward. It was approximately nine hours after I had reported to the ER initially. The nurse who admitted me to the ward asked me similar questions like those in the ER, but he also wrote that I slept with the TENS machine on. I immediately asked for a pillow to elevate my injured leg, which should have been given to me since I was in the ER. In the ward, the doctor ordered antibiotics, on IV piggyback, along with NS (normal saline) at 75 cc an hour, with leg-compression hoses. That was an ideal order for shock and, at the same time, for protecting my heart from pericarditis because of my history of cardiac disease.

They brought my PO (by mouth) medication, and as I inquired what it was, I found out that it included Synthroid as well. The Synthroid was the reason that brought on the shaking in the first place, and this is a very good example of misdiagnosed problems. Everyone placed emphasis on the left ankle ulcer but ignored the initial shaking/trembling, which was most likely due to the overdose of Synthroid over time. So I refused to take the Synthroid, and the doctor finally discontinued the Synthroid.

The body has a built-in mechanism to handle shock. There are three stages of shock: the initial one is compensation, which, if not treated, can quickly lead to the second stage of tachycardia with hypotension. I think, but I have no evidence, that my TSH went below zero value during that day, and I developed a fever and the body compensated to drive the TSH up to 0.56. I am a brittle diabetic, so I had my glucose checked every four hours. I also now appreciate the disgust that patients endure when awakening them every four hours.

The next morning, blood was sent to the lab, and there was evidence of an infection. That day they changed me from Zosyn, after having had three doses, to Levaquin—three doses every eight hours. The second night after admission, I was awakened at 0315h by three frantic nurses and two nurses' aids.

I was kept on my usual diabetic medication of metformin and glyburide, but my glucose was still covered with insulin. They informed me that my glucose level was at 44. Usually, if my glucose drops below 60, my eyes become blurry, my heart rate increases, and I feel very sleepy; but there were not any such symptoms. I drank four small boxes of orange juice, and my glucose increased to 85. That pleased them, and I returned to sleep only to be awakened at 0400h for regular repeating blood draws. The next morning, the doctor (resident) visited and was told about the decreased glucose incident. He showed some anger, and I guess that it was the intern who wrote the orders that included metformin, glyburide, and insulin. The metformin and glyburide were discontinued, and a sliding scale for insulin was written.

Then he noticed that my feet were swollen and the thrombo embolic deterrent (TED) hoses were not on. He insisted that the nurse place them on immediately, and the swelling disappeared in 24 hours. I was lucky that I had a nurse who knew how to place TED hoses on without hurting me. If he reads this book, I thank him very much. I did eventually mention this to the ward's head nurse. I was given Dilaudid a narcotic intravenously every four hours, and that regimen seemed to control my right shoulder pain. Many thanks to the doctors who ordered it and to the nurses that dispensed it willingly. It's amazing that without looking at the clock, I knew I needed that medication every four hours. I had no problem getting it on time.

The next night, I went to the bathroom (toilet), and when I returned, I had an attack like asthma; I could hardly breathe. I told the nurse, and she said that it was because I sprayed Lysol around the phone and room. I always spray my phone with Lysol and around all my rooms at home. I immediately thought of fluid overload. I was receiving NS at 75 cc an hour, since admission, and I had already received 5-250 cc antibiotic boluses, and I was on an 1800-cal diet. I asked her to call the doctor and ask for a respiratory breathing treatment; after a little convincing, she finally complied.

I received a treatment of albuterol with Atrovent, and the IV was reduced to 15 cc an hour. I felt relieved almost immediately. If this nurse had read my history, she would have recognized the signs and symptoms of fluid overload. I was also on Demadex (toresemide) at home (a potent diuretic—which I never received from the time I entered up to discharge). The next day, I thought I felt a little better and spoke with the intern. The swelling of my feet was reducing, and I felt I should go home. I was more terrified of what they may do to me; more importantly, I had to insist that everyone flushing my IV flush the air out of the syringe. No nurse removed the air unless I asked them to do so. This is considered a major error as it only takes 0.5 cc of air to cause an embolus.

It really scared me to know that they flushed IVs and Heparin locks (heplocks) without discarding the air out of the prefilled syringe. A heplock is an IV that has been capped and is not hocked up to any fluid. It is called a heplock because previously in the 1980's, all heplocks were flushed every four hours with heparin. After many trials it was discovered that normal saline does the same job of maintaining patency in the heplock. After about a day, those who flushed my IV made it into a joke that they were discarding the air out of the syringe; however, I can deal with the jokes versus my life. It would only take about one to two cc of air to form a pulmonary embolus (PE). Very importantly, the intern ripped my compressing socks down to inspect my ankle, and that really hurt. I can safely say that intern never had the experience of putting on or taking off compression stockings.

My IV on the right hand was changed by a registered nurse, whom I recognized as one that I oriented and trained in the ICU when he was an LVN (licensed practical nurse); the supervisor recommended him after I requested that the anesthesia reps restart my IVs. When he saw me, he immediately boasted about what a good nursing instructor I was, and I almost felt embarrassed at his excellent announcements. I thought that this would be the test of how well I had taught him. Fortunately, he got the IV with his first and only stick. I really thanked him, but he was thanking me even more for all that I taught him.

I never saw the intern again, but the staff doctor and the resident were discussing my case at the bedside the next morning and referring to me in the third person. I intimated that my hemoglobin/hematocrit was low at 10/30—usually it was at about 14/42. The staff doctor immediately said that it was because of hemodilution, but the blood was drawn in the ER before any administration of any fluid, so it couldn't be from hemodilution. This is the guessing game I spoke about earlier. On that note, I decided that I needed to get out of this hospital. I was given one dose of vancomycin at 700 mg. Blood was drawn, and I know that the trough was low. So I was given two doses of 1,000-mg vancomycin in eight hours and finally discharged. My wife took me home with tablets of Zosyn and doxycycline.

Hypothyroidism was never addressed. I should note that I never saw any doctor or nurse wash their hands before and after they came into my room. I now think that it is important to show the patient that you have washed your hands. Hand washing is the very basic concept of maintaining a safe and sterile environment.

AT HOME

As soon as I returned home, I took the diuretic (Demadex), and that reduced my fluid status considerably. Apparently, that hospital does not have Demadex in pill form. I was really relived that I was back home, and if I died, that's where I wanted to be. I slept like a "baby," but I had very strange dreams about Iraq and Saddam. I dreamed that I was in an antimatter clinic, and I had the capability of dissipating all material in that clinic with the flick of a finger. I understood in the dream that the purpose of that building was to destroy all of Saddam's oil dealings with the West and how he had kept it a secret for so long.

I was discharged on Tuesday, and by Friday, I took my blood sugar. It was exceedingly high, with a value of 280, and I became very concerned. I concluded that the antibiotics that I was given had been infused too fast and in too short of time between administration intervals.

A LITTLE KNOWLEDGE
CAN BE A BAD THING

I was very, very weak. I had to hold on to my wife, or the walls, in order to navigate to the bathroom. My first stool was black, and I flushed it down quickly; I didn't want to see it as it most likely meant that I was bleeding in my stomach or intestines. I didn't tell my wife but contemplated what would eventually occur. I thought that the supposed bleeding was caused by my liver and that my glucose was so high because of my pancreas. I thought that, from experience, if my liver and pancreas was failing, the next organ to go would be my kidneys. These thoughts rested with me continuously.

My wife and I went outside, and she intimated that I was getting better, but I felt otherwise. On Saturday I had called the resident and intimated the value of my glucose. He had replied that it was not an emergency, that I didn't have to report to the ER, but I could take an extra glyburide. I had done as he recommended, but the glucose had only been reduced to 240. I had called him again on Sunday and almost insisted that he see me and address this glucose increase, so he had suggested that I see him on Monday morning. This had relieved my fears slightly; I still had not mentioned anything about having black stool. I thought that finally I would be bleeding through my esophagus and that after banding by a gastroenterologist, they would be unable to stop the bleeding and I would be intubated, placed on a ventilator, finally be made a DNR (do not resuscitate), and die. I was really preparing myself for this.

My wife said that I was uttering some sentences that sounded as if I was a little disoriented. I eventually built up some courage and asked her to look at my stool, and she replied that it looked like the remnants of broccoli; this felt like a weight off my chest, for I knew that I had eaten broccoli in the hospital. But I was still convinced that there was something wrong with my liver and pancreas, for I now felt very weak and couldn't think very clearly. I also was not eating and not hungry, and most diabetics don't miss a meal.

On Monday morning, I visited the hospital and spoke with the resident on the phone. He suggested that I wait until after he had completed rounds, and then, somehow, he'd work me into his clinic. In the meantime I went to my usual blood-drawing clinic, and they readily drew my blood. The order was placed for November, but somehow they did not question the urgency. Then I went to my doctor's office and asked if I could see him. There I was told that I still had time to report in sick. I was not familiar with these regulations, but I did write my name down for a sick call. After about half an hour, I was called into an office by a registered nurse. I intimated what had occurred and pointed out that my glucose was elevated. She asked me what I wanted her to do—what a question from a registered nurse—but I replied, "Tell the doctor." I was really expecting him to start me on insulin.

Well, she finally returned and said that the doctor wanted a finger stick, something she should have done initially, to check my glucose level. She tested my glucose, and showed me the meter read the level as 120; I knew immediately that my glucometer at home was incorrect. I could have jumped for joy at this news. I visited the ICU and immediately retested my glucose at work, and it was 130; I could live with that difference figuratively, but this confirmed that I was not hyperglycemic. I had already worked out how my illness would progress and how I'd die. The doctor, however, pointed out that my lab results were back and that my ammonia was high at 43. This confirmed my suspicion that my liver had an insult from the harsh antibiotics and, most likely, the speed with which they had been given. I continued taking the antibiotics that I was given to take at home, but after five days, I stopped because of really severe diarrhea. It took me one month to be able to drive and ambulate without any help. I had lost forty pounds.

I returned to work, and I couldn't believe the great reception that I received. I worked for three days at that department and was taken personally to the administration floor by my senior supervisor, where I was tasked with the job of preparing a two-day course for nursing assistants. But I felt so weak that I knew that the time had arrived for me to retire. I was already sixty-two years old, had served twenty-seven years up, my right shoulder was not getting any better and I had worked fifteen years after having open heart bypass surgery. I had seen all the doctors that I thought could help with diagnosis and repair, but without relief.

After retirement, I inadvertently came across an ad on a herb for arthritis; I bought it and used it. After three weeks, I awoke one morning and noticed that there was something strange with my body: the right shoulder pain had dissipated, thank GOD. I could not truly attribute this healing to this herb or that it healed all by itself, but I'm glad that it's gone. I never got that pain again.

So to recap what can be learned from this excursion:

1. Neither the doctor nor the nurse listened carefully to me, the patient.
2. The source of the ulcer, decreased TSH, was never addressed, and if I didn't refuse the Synthroid that night, I would have been shaking again as if I had Parkinson's.
3. The doctor's order (compression stockings) was not obeyed; it was on the nurses' orders that they pulled up from the computer every shift, and all ignored it. I would have liked to see what orders they were signing off in the computer as "given."
4. If the nurse had read my history and noted my symptoms, she would have known that if hot versus cold is involved, suspect the thyroid. So I question the administration of more Synthroid.
5. The necessity of introducing an IV was immediate; being without an IV for 5 hours in the ER is inexcusable, especially when the patient shows the first sign of shock.
6. The intern should have been aware of the effects of diabetes medication (pills) with the action of insulin, but the nurses should have brought the conflicting orders to the doctor too.
7. The antibiotics were given at too close of intervals and were probably infused too fast.

8. The nurse should have been able to recognize fluid overload, even by reading the history and physical. At least listen to the patient's lungs and heart. More importantly always listen to your patient, for the patient knows his or her body more than anyone, especially if the patient was an ICU nurse.

9. This intern should try on one of the embolic stockings to know how it feels and how gently he should pull it down. It really hurt because the legs were red, hot, tender and there was an open ulcer present. May I use the word "*empathy*"?

10. Demadex should have been ordered on admission and given as I said I had a history of congestive heart failure (CHF).

11. There was no washing of hands on entry or exit of my room.

12. I was discharged without any mention or address of hypothyroidism.

13. These are all errors that could be avoided, and my aim is not to embarrass anyone but to let others be cognizant of these errors. Perhaps readers will not commit the same errors.

My next example will make your skin shiver as I unveil gross inefficiency and, perhaps, what can be considered malpractice. Please read on. I have tried to state these facts with the most forthright euphemisms available in my diction; it is not my intention to anger anyone or distort any of the stated facts. The next example will surely blow your mind.

INEFFICIENCY VERSUS MALPRACTICE

I had just reported for duty at 1445h and was told that I would be getting a post-op (postoperative) patient, a hernia repair. Today, hernia repairs are considered simple, not-so-dangerous operations. However, even as I say this, the administration of anesthesia is just as much or more dangerous than the actual operation. As I was preparing the room for the post-op patient, someone rolled a RotoRest bed into the room. The saleswoman/coordinator of that company was present. I had read about these beds being excellent for ARDS (acute respiratory distress syndrome), but our hospital did not have one. This demonstration that the representative was going to perform was going to be treated as in-service. This smelled fishy to me because I now understood that the post-op patient was going to be on this bed, so I'd better learn the operation quickly.

This bed, even though effective for the physical treatment of ARDS and the prevention of decubitus (a bed sore), would be very terrifying for a conscious patient. There is a mask that is placed over the patient's face, and the whole front of the body is covered. The bed is then rotated over, placing the patient on the stomach, rotating at whatever angle that the operator sets. The aim is to keep the patient off the back and, at the same time, rotate left and right. Sedation is necessary and the bed should be stopped, the patient placed on the back, and all equipment placed in front of the patient removed to enable a thorough examination of the patient. There are standing orders written as to how often this should be done.

ARDS can be treated with high peep (pulmonary end expiratory pressure) given by a ventilator, while the patient is sedated and monitored meticulously for barotrauma per SOP (standard operating procedures). The aim is recruitment of the alveoli by keeping them open so as to absorb the maximum of oxygen possible. I am not giving an in-service on ARDS, but some of the causes are

- Pneumonia
- drowning
- ventilator-assisted pneumonia
- long periods of intubation in the OR
- multiple organ dysfunction

In the middle of this in service on the RotoRest bed, my patient arrived, intubated and sedated. My voluntary team and I went to work, placing the patient on the RotoRest bed. Her oxygen saturation (SO2) by pulse oximeter was at 80 percent—this is considered critical. The bed representative promised that her respiratory function would improve as soon as we turned her on her stomach. Lo and behold, she was correct; as soon as we turned her, the oxygen saturation increased to 97 percent. It took about a good half hour with five volunteer nurses and I to fit all the pieces and IV and arterial lines in place.

The history of this patient was that she had had a hernia repair by laparotomy and was sent home the same day, but returned the next because of severe abdominal pain. She was treated with Tylenol and sent back home. She returned the following day complaining of severe excruciating pain and was finally taken to the OR, where she had an open abdominal exploration. There was evidence of peritonitis. The abdomen was washed and cleaned, the puncture was repaired, and her abdomen was stapled together for closure.

She rested that night, sedated. We occasionally placed her on her back and removed the front of the bed with the mask to examine her status physically. I spoke to her during the night while I checked the tubing of the IVs and the ventilator. She was very comfortable, and I could ascertain this by her heart rate, blood pressure, oximeter reading, respirations, and urine output. I took care of her for the next two nights, but realized that she had a high temperature, her blood pressure was lower than usual, and tachycardia was present. I intimated to the doctors that there was something not right with this patient. She had diarrhea, most likely from the antibiotics, but her abdomen was a little distended.

The next morning, I prepared her for surgery (pre-op), and they promptly wheeled her off to the OR for another open abdominal exploratory operation. The results were alarming, for in their previous closure the abdomen wall was stapled together and had somehow involved the intestines. You may say that the intestines were stapled to the inner abdomen. This would surely again cause peritonitis as the contents of the intestines leaked into the perineum. They, the surgeons, again washed out the abdomen and stapled her up.

By this time she was off the ventilator, on a mask, and was alert after the operation. She was still kept on pain medication and was comfortable until, two days later, she again showed signs of infection and pain.

In the meantime, I developed a great trust with this patient and her family. I involved the mother in bathing her and making her comfortable. Everyone concerned said that we had "bonded"; the mother and husband asked that the management detail me to look after her exclusively. This was a little impossible, or highly improbable, as there were other patients in the ICU who needed my expertise. I think that my voice, my maturity, and the confidence I portrayed was responsible for this "bonding." I still followed her progress and I know that she had to be taken again to the OR for the same signs and symptoms, but this time another team performed the intervention. That was the last operation she had for that year; it was finally corrected.

Because of the length of stay with multiple nurses and doctors in and out of her room, handling her dressing/feedings, she developed multiple "bugs" at various stages of her care. She developed hospital-acquired MRSA (methicillin-resistant *Staphylococcus aureus*); a terrible bug to cure. So occasionally, I still took care of her, and I thought that her confidence in me started while she was sedated but could somehow remember my voice.

This really is a very good example of gross incompetence and neglect. I know that she was about to sue, but they settled for a large sum of compensation. If ever I am sick, I would like that group of surgeons to stay far away from my door. I used to joke that if ever I have to be hospitalized, I have a list of nurses who may take care of or even visit me. The above example surely requires someone with medical knowledge to follow the patient's condition and care. Not everyone has been created equal. As an example, there are good plumbers, excellent plumbers, bad plumbers and worst plumbers, likewise there are excellent nurses and doctors, good nurses and doctors, bad nurses and doctors and worse nurses and doctors. That is a fact.

I was called by my name one morning about four years ago, as I entered the hospital, by a young female, and I inquired if she knew me. It was the same patient that I bonded with, and she intimated that she was going to have a repeat of the same surgery by laparotomy the next day. I never saw her in the ICU, so I can conclude that it went okay. What an ordeal it must have been for this young lady and her family. Terror can be the least description that fits her visit to the hospital.

CRITICAL AND ALMOST
FATAL ERROR

I had reported for duty one evening and was receiving reports from the previous charge nurse when we were abruptly interrupted by calls for help from several nurses. There was a code blue on the ICU unit. I was charge nurse for that evening. There was a nurse who had initially belonged to a step-down ICU and who had been oriented on the ICU twice. I am not going to comment on the orientation, but when I orient anyone on the ICU, I start as if they are not aware of any of our tasks, skills, or responsibilities.

There was a shift that was referred to as a fourth shift for slightly injured/sick nurses. This shift usually started at 10:00 a.m. and ended at 1800h. So it embedded both the first and second shifts. As I entered the ICU that evening, I met this nurse who was always pleasant to me. She had been a registered nurse for many years, had BCLS (basic cardiac life support) and ACLS (advanced cardiac life support). I have been an instructor of ACLS for at least eighteen years. I asked her what her assignment was, and she replied that she had ended up watching four patients as the nurses taking care of those patients were either at dinner or had gone to the bathroom.

As I was receiving report on all the patients in the unit, code blue was sounded, both the previous charge nurse and I ran to the ICU floor. CPR was in progress. I saw that the patient was in asystole (flatline rhythm) on the cardiac monitor. We started using epinephrine (which acts as a vasodilator/ pressor) and the patient's heart rhythm would return to a sinus block, but it also returned an asystolic state. Atropine was used, but the main rhythm remained asystolic until the nurse who was watching the patient confessed that she had made a mistake and gave the patient 250 cc of fentanyl, an opioid used for controlling severe pain.

The doctor, a pulmonologist, immediately ordered Narcan, and after several doses, the patient returned to a sinus rhythm with occasional premature ventricular contractions (PVC). The patient continued to return to a sinus rhythm but would convert back to other unacceptable heart rhythms. CPR was always initiated on seeing this disorder until finally a steady pulse was recognized. A Narcan drip was ordered and started. The patient was now intubated and remained the night in the ICU. She was extubated the following day and, after spending another night, was sent to the ward/floor.

I had to write an incident report and also give my recommendations. I discovered that this error had evolved from a doctor's verbal order to give 250 cc of saline because of a urine output below 30 cc in one hour.

This patient had been extubated the day before this incident and had orders to be moved to the ward/floor. The patient had been receiving fentanyl while she was intubated. The fentanyl had been discontinued, but the tubing was not removed from the IV. At the same time, another tube had been running normal saline through her IV at 15 cc an hour so as to keep the vein open and offer slight hydration. The nurse had checked but had failed to recognize that the pump she initiated was fentanyl and not saline. The strength of fentanyl in the ICU is 10 mcg per cc, so this patient had been given 250 cc by 10, which equals to 2,500 cc of fentanyl in about fifteen minutes (a bolus). That had caused the patient to stop breathing. This patient had been extremely lucky that the monitor alarms were on, and we were lucky that the right doctor and the right nurses were present and that the nurse involved quickly admitted that she had erred. I would like to emphasize the need for setting alarms and paying attention to detail. A patient in the ICU most likely would have several IV solutions running concurrently. These IV lines must be labeled and traced physically to ensure that it is the right IV line you intend to employ.

I would like to come to the defense of this nurse, although it is inexcusable to commit such an error that almost ended in fatal results. That fourth shift is so designed that the nurse ends up helping others around the unit. That shift does not accommodate the nurse taking care of a specific patient, and often many nurses take advantage of this extra body. This nurse—no nurse—can adequately take care of four sick ICU patients without sacrificing some care. So my recommendations were that this shift be discontinued but that the nurse should have implemented the five rights of medications, and they are

1. to ensure that it is the right patient and doctor,
2. to ensure that the diagnosis is right and that the drug is for that diagnosis,
3. to ensure that the right dose is correct,
4. to ensure that the right route is correct,
5. to ensure that the speed of infusion is correct, and
6. to ensure that you know the side effects of the drug and the compatibility with other drugs.

Chart that the drug was given, assess, and evaluate. You can't go too far wrong with this method. This nurse, I am sure, knew all the rights of giving medication but was overloaded with orders and caring for four patients. The nurse resigned, but the administration should take a little blame too, from the top to the bottom. Surely it was by the grace of God and the expertise of those involved that there had been a good ending.

POINTS TO NOTE

Always know your limits; do not try to be a superman or a superwoman when lives are involved. If you ever feel pressured, speak out, beg, or complain. Remember and implement the five rights of giving medication. There is no *best nurse*; you are only so good because of help from your peers. No one knows everything; if you don't know, ask/find out. Offer solutions to reflect that you are not uncooperative but that as soon as one of the nurses returns from dinner, you'll be glad to take care of others.

There is always the tendency to accept and not deny the wishes of others, especially if you are in that team. This can be detrimental to the care and excellent nursing in a team. The team is only as strong as the weakest link, and those who are stronger and are team leaders must possess the insight on the capability of the team and not only join the ride.

THE OTHER SIDE OF THE COIN

This happens to be the true name of the book, but I purposely added *medical* to the name of this book so as to draw the attention of doctors, nurses, and patients. As a teenager, I thought I was gung ho, meaning that I thought there were no limits to my capability. My culture prevented me from showing much emotion and not to cry even at funerals or if I was in great pain. I remember when, while playing soccer, I fell and my knees dragged on the sand, causing terrible burning painful "road rash." I did not cry, but I went to the medic who immediately said, "You are going to bawl for this is going to burn and hurt." He proceeded to introduce/paint my skinless knees with iodine. There are no words in the dictionary that can adequately express how terrible the burning I felt from that iodine was. I tried to imagine that I was in a better place, and I acknowledged that this was my punishment for some of my sins and that I must bear it. I had to wear short pants for three weeks.

Another time, I was riding my racing bicycle and the generator that I had affixed to the front fork rolled down into the spokes. The generator was put on for night riding and also offered some resistance so that my muscles could get stronger for future racing. I emphasize *racing* because you can imagine how fast I was going. The front wheel locked immediately, and I was thrown above the handle of the bike for about twenty feet onto the surface of a tarmac road, face-first. I can't remember getting up, so I must have blacked out. But when I was finally on my feet, I looked up and saw a girl at the window of a house, and I recognized her as a pupil of the same school I attended. I asked her if I could have some water, and she said there was a pipe in the yard. I washed my face, which was completely numb, and I asked her to convey to my teacher the reason for my absence.

The bike was so mangled that it was impossible to ride. I was about four blocks from home, so I lifted my bicycle on my shoulder and made my way home. I was taken to the doctor and the same treatment was meted out, except this time I was given pain medication. So in all the above, I intended to accentuate the no-crying culture, but I don't condemn those who do cry—perhaps only in my little twisted mind.

I was enlisted in the American army at the age of thirty-four years old, considered old for doing basic training; but I had already passed through this training many times before, so I knew what to expect, what to do, and what not to do—and I was very fit. I could run faster and longer than any instructor—actually, I was more educated than most of the instructors. My GCE certificates were accepted as a high school diploma, but I had already done advanced English literature and advanced mathematics. I completed that basic course with a hernia—the dangerous effects of which I now know of—but I had to pass.

During my soldering career in the United States Army, I felt numbness in my arms, fingers, and occasionally in my chest. The first doctor I saw for this complaint diagnosed it as carpal tunnel syndrome. He was an ear, nose, and throat doctor "pulling call." As time progressed, I found out that my cholesterol and triglycerides were high. I received minimal treatment for this, and there was no significant follow-up. My EKG (electrocardiogram) showed that my RS was depressed, and I was given a stress test. I ran for twenty minutes on the treadmill, and the MICU (medical intensive care unit) doctor concluded that my heart was in perfect working order. My cholesterol remained elevated, but I was given orders to go to Germany. I then started to feel chest pains in Germany, and I had another stress test. I ran for twelve minutes on the treadmill, and the test was terminated because of no chest pain. There were other things I did in Germany that I am not going to get into here.

I was transferred to Fort Ord, and this time I knew that what I was feeling as I did physical training was real chest pain. I reported sick twice, and the first time, I saw a PA (physician's assistant). I brought to his attention that my ST segment was depressed and my T wave was inverted. By this time I was an ACLS instructor. This jackass (and I hope he is reading this book) said to me that 75 percent of the people in the United States have EKGs just like mine. This, he intimated, was normal and nothing was wrong with me. My next visit to sick call, I saw a doctor who was more interested in sticking his finger in my ass than addressing my chest pain. This really made me question the competency of these doctors. I also was sent to a rheumatologist for chest pain.

The chest pain continued as I exerted myself, and I remembered three noncommissioned officers at different intervals of time falling dead in another army that I was in, after (or during) running six miles with full kit. My duty fulfillment was almost up, and after pleading with my commander (and I sincerely thank him for that), I was given an honorable discharge. I worked at a trauma center ICU in California for about a year, but because of my wife, who was also an ICU nurse, could not stand the earth tremors, we moved to another state.

I was employed in the SICU (surgical intensive care unit), and this was my final dream. I wanted to know more and more about surgical procedures and how to care for surgical patients. We had open-heart patients on the unit, and as I passed them, I thought that this was one type of operation I could do without. However, I still had occasional chest pain and dismissed it as normal. This time I did not want to face the reality that it could be a blockage of an artery. I did report to the ER at least twice for chest pain, but my enzymes and my EKG, except for the depressed ST segment, were normal. These are still classic signs of a heart blockage and should have been followed more aggressively.

Then one day I was sent home early, working eight instead of twelve hours, and as I exited the hospital, I felt chest pain and a more severe numbness in my upper arms and fingers. I knew the signs and symptoms fitted a heart attack and that I should visit the ER, but I was really hoping foolishly that it would dissipate on its own. I was in full blown denial. I arrived home by driving and sat on my sofa. I knew that if it was a blockage that my heart was not getting the required amount of oxygen and that if I moved, exerted myself, my heart would need even more oxygen. I still teach that maneuver today. If chest pain and numbness of the arms, hands, and back of neck are present, stay still but call 911 (for an ambulance).

I waited for about twenty minutes, and my wife arrived home. I immediately asked her to take me to the ER. In the ER, again my enzymes were normal, but there was enough abnormality on my EKG for the doctor to order a stress test via a cardiologist. I was distraught; the doctor wanted to admit me, but I denied him and went home. There was no further chest pain that night. What I may add is that I had chest pain and arm numbness all the way to the hospital, but as soon as I was placed on the gurney of the hospital, the pain left. At that time, I felt foolish as the doctor asked me, "Where is the pain?" and I said, "It's gone." But for those who do not know, such reactions are very common. It almost seemed as if I was using personification, as if this pain had its own life. I thought that for once I had seen a doctor who was not taking any chances.

The next morning I visited the cardiologist, and he felt there might not be anything wrong, because of my age and fitness, but went ahead and started the stress test. Less than two minutes into the test, I felt that same chest pain. The cardiologist stopped the test and sprayed nitroglycerin under my tongue. The pain immediately subsided. The cardiologist felt that I may have only one blockage and it may be in the circumflex artery. He scheduled a coronary catheterization for the following Monday. The day of the stress test was Friday.

Most doctors felt that because I was in my forties, it could not be my heart. I was and looked very fit at that time. My father had passed in February that same year, (may he rest in peace), and it was now April. Some of this may be attributed to stress, but I knew that with high cholesterol and triglycerides and WBCs (white blood cells) always slightly elevated, there was a blockage somewhere.

So here I am awaiting a cardiac catheterization, lying almost naked on the table, when the doctor arrived. I had an IV and 2 mg (milligrams) of Versed was introduced. As the doctor felt for the femoral artery, I may have moved, because I heard him say, "Give two more milligrams of Versed." That knocked me out completely (put me to sleep). The next thing I heard was the cardiologist awakening me and saying that there were 90 percent blockages in the LAD (left anterior descending) artery and the RCA (right coronary artery) and its branches, and that he recommended heart bypass surgery. I remember that moment so vividly, as if it were yesterday. I was awake but drowsy, but I heard and understood his statement completely. I knew what it meant.

I felt as if the bed had opened up and I had fallen six feet down into the earth; in a matter of seconds, my life had turned upside down. Now it was not a simple hernia, of which I had been operated on three times, but this operation included stopping my heart to have it repaired. It's rerouting the plumbing of my coronary system; what if they couldn't restart my heart? The cardiac surgeon uses very small Paddles to give a jolt to the heart and usually it restarts. What if the PA allows air into the pump and is unable to prime it out? How skillful is the anesthesiologist, and how many cases has he done? Why would God do this to me? I help people live.

Then I thought of all those sins I had committed and of how I thought that if I loaded them up in a bag, I wouldn't be able to lift that bag. All these questions and answers flew through my mind in a matter of seconds. Then I thought, *I am still sleepy, and I'll sleep. I'll deal with the consequences later.* They wheeled me out to post-op, placed a ten-pound sandbag on my right groin, and I went back to sleep.

I was later awakened by the technician, who brought the pictures of the blockages to show me. I couldn't really focus on them, and I went back to sleep. She came three distinct times, but somehow, as she turned the machine, I couldn't focus on the blockages—all looked the same to me. Then came the cardiac surgeon; my wife knew him as she had worked for him occasionally in the past. I knew him, but except for saying good morning, he and I had not had any real conversations. I always wondered how he could fit his huge, fat, stumpy fingers into patients' chests. They were twice the size of mine, and he was not as tall as I.

He intimated that I needed cardiac surgery emergently. He really caught me off guard, so I asked him what he was going to do. I was hoping he'd tell me in great detail, prolong the conversation, and give me time to think. He was ready to wheel me into surgery immediately. I told him I didn't know what the surgery was all about, and could I do without it. This seemed to anger him as he raised his voice and said that I was an RN and I should know what he was talking about. Well, surely, I knew what he was saying, but I was hoping for a little more rapport to build my confidence that everything was going to be okay. More so, I was playing for time to think.

I got to know him better later on because I took care of his patients, and he pointed me out as an example of his good work. After the IV was removed and the sandbag was taken away, I finally sent for him and requested that the operation be done on Monday, three days away. He agreed and I went home; I had to conserve all my energies and prepare myself mentally for this ordeal. I knew what they did, and I was aware of the postoperative care that was given. I knew there was rehab and that I would be off work for some time.

On Sunday, my brother-in-law picked me up in his car, and we went to the casino. On the way back, I felt chest pain, so I took a tablet of nitroglycerin under my tongue. I felt really bad and began to perspire; immediately, I thought that my blood pressure was low (hypotension). I intimated to my brother-in-law how I felt, but instead of driving me straight home, he took me into the army base where he bought bread because it was about three cents cheaper than the commercial bakeries outside. There was nothing that I could do except keep my feet elevated and the back of the chair retracted. I was taken home and my wife and I had a good laugh, but I still kept my feet higher than my heart. This seemed to return my body to normal hemostasis. My daughter visited, and I was very glad she did, but I don't think she knew the magnitude of the operation or disease. She was still in primary school.

THE PREPARATION AND
THE OPERATION

I spent that Sunday night at home but reported to the hospital at 0200h on Monday morning. That was the last time I smoked a cigarette, and never again craved it or had any withdrawal symptoms. If it's called "cold turkey," then that's what I did. I have always been able to turn on or off my habits and desires with due diligence. I reported to the emergency room the Monday morning and was sent up to a single room where I met a nurse and a respiratory technician.

The nurse took scant information, and the respiratory tech did an arterial puncture for a blood-gas baseline. My paO_2 was 60, barely making the grade to generate a SaO_2 of 90 percent. These numbers bothered me a little, but the tech kept me talking while she meticulously shaved me from neck to ankle. We spoke about chest tubes and how many I would recover on completion of the operation.

I saw the doctor who initially suggested a stress test, and after I announced what the results were and that I was going to have surgery, he said, "Well, you have youth on your side." Usually most, except a very minor few, who have had this operation were at least sixty years old. This statement by that doctor offered some comfort. So after the shaving, I was given an antimicrobial soap and asked to scrub my skin thoroughly. After drying, I returned to the bed as naked as when I was born, and that disturbed me a little. The waiting was the longest that I have ever experienced, but all fear had, by now, left my senses.

At about 830 A.M. I was wheeled in and placed in front of the OR area. I even intimated to the nurse that I had not signed an anesthesia form, which basically says that if you need blood, it is okay to give you some and that this operation may consist of bleeding and may even terminate in *death*. When they brought it, I signed it. At this time, I think my wife was more worried than I was. All fear had left me, and as they wheeled me into the OR, I kept saying or arguing with myself that I should not be afraid because this was where I worked. I knew these machines, sounds and instruments. This was a huge contrast to my second hernia operation. At that time I was fifteen years old and as the porters (they were called in those days) wheeled me to the OR, I got off the gurney and tried to run away. The porters caught up with me and escorted me back and placed me on the gurney. I did not have the right of free choice in those days, in an underdeveloped country. I had the operation performed on me that day.

I slid over to the operating slab, holding the sheet between my legs, but I knew that they would soon remove it as soon as I was sedated. I knew that they would insert a Foley into my bladder, but as soon as I was on the slab, the PA started working on an arterial line. I did not feel very much pain, which says she was very skilled. The anesthetist was talking to me all the time, asked about where I worked and also started an IV. Then I was asleep/sedated and most likely paralyzed.

The next thing I can remember was a friend/peer from work waking me with a very loud voice. He said, "It's over, the operation is over. You're all right." I remember well that I was intubated, bilaterally restrained, and could not move a muscle, except my eyes. I could blink. I wanted to work out a sign language of my eyes with him, but I think he was more overjoyed than I. I knew I was alive, and I knew that I couldn't use my arms and legs because the paralytic, probably narcuron or sacs, was still in my system. If I was not an SICU nurse, I would have freaked out, but I knew that with time the effects would wear off. But I tried my best with my greatest effort, and I moved my left foot once. I returned to sleep as I heard them say they were leaving. It is not a real nice feeling to open your eyes and you cannot move your limbs. I can also remember the nurse that accepted me out of the OR say that I was on my back all the time and that she needed to turn me. She asked if I would pull anything if she released one hand. I shook my hand; I was too scared to move my head knowing that I was intubated. I knew they would know when to extubate me, but If I accidently extubated myself, it could be disastrous.

Around ten p.m. another nurse that took over and told me that I was ready for extubation, so she also called the respiratory tech. But she threw saline down my endotracheal tube—a big no-no in the ICU. I started coughing and couldn't stop. I looked up at the heart monitor and saw my heart rate had jumped up to 220 beats a minute. I knew she was also scared, for when the tech asked her if she was ready, she replied to wait until my heart rate returned to normal. I felt as if I was drowning, but I still kept my hands to my side; for if I had only moved them above my abdomen, she may have restrained them again.

Finally I was extubated and could talk. I emphatically told her without any hesitation that nurses don't throw saline down endotracheal tubes anymore, especially when the patient was very alert. There were articles printed on this subject and one of the questions that arose was, what happens to the saline that is delivered to the lungs via the endotracheal tube when the suction catheter does not suck out any fluid?

Also bacteria in the endotracheal tube will be forced down into the lungs with the introduction of saline. She replied that she was not aware of that fact, so I said, "Take this as an in-service on suctioning." Usually before suctioning a patient's lungs, you should listen before and after.

There was nothing in my lungs for her to suction. I didn't see any nurse listen to my lungs or heart from admission to discharge. I asked for food, and the nurse said that I should try ice first. I insisted that I eat food but that she could bring the ice, and I was also willing to demonstrate that I could swallow and keep it down. She brought a small TV dinner, and I think I gobbled it down. Then I spoke with my wife, who I thought was very tired and sleepy. I remained in ICU for about four days, during which I had several nurses.

There was a code blue in the room next to mine on the next day, Tuesday, and everyone—I mean, everyone—was in there. There was no one looking at the other patients. I had a nurse one morning, who I had worked with before since we were both LVNs at that time. We were both ICU RNs now. She and my wife had had an altercation because someone had let my wife in the ICU without her permission. She was not examining me, or doing anything very important, and she also knew my wife, so I thought this gung ho bit was a form of a little Caesar syndrome. I saw this nurse at 7 a.m. and again at 3 p.m., then she started apologizing for her neglect. I just let it go, but did not think very much of her nursing ability. I still say hi to her anytime I see her. I would really like to see what she charted on me—perhaps that I am still alive? Or stable, no complaints of any problems? I am sure that she knows that I know that she didn't do a good job. I didn't have a bath of any cleaning for 5 days.

I did not mention that I had an NG tube, a Foley, and three chest tubes—two bilateral and one epigastric. I remember that every time the ventilator gave me a breath, the epigastric chest tube area hurt terribly, but I never complained. I was given Toradol every eight hours. As they changed the ventilator settings from SIMV to pressure support only, I could feel that I was breathing much better. I can advise nurses who have patients with a Foley the following:

1. Don't raise the Foley above the pelvic region.
2. Don't leave the Foley unsecured to the skin.
3. Don't move the Foley very quickly, for it feels as if it's wiggling in your bladder.
4. Observe for stricture problems.
5. Tape the foley above the pelvis or the patient can have stricture problems.

The third-day post-op, I had to go to the bathroom. I requested a commode and not a bed pan. This was real arduous work, transporting my chest tube bottles onto one side of the bed. I had a tiny bowel movement, but that really gave me a lot of relief. I am truly grateful for them, the nurses, for assisting me in getting on that commode without any comments.

The next day, the cardiac surgeon came to pull the chest tubes. I was terrified, and it might have showed. He ordered 1 mg morphine to be given SQ (subcutaneously); I don't think that did very much for my anxiety. I have seen patients in the ICU shout out in pain as the chest tube is removed. Finally, all my chest tubes were removed, and all I felt was a little tickle at the site. Only a master can remove chest tubes with such ease. I was later transferred to a step-down unit. I had a private room, and I was grateful for that. Visitors were in and out.

The first night in the step-down unit, I was awakened by the respiratory technician. He tested my oxygen saturation by placing an oximeter on my finger, and it read 88 percent. He seemed as if he was scared and said to me that he was going to call the doctor. He returned and placed a nasal cannula on, with oxygen at two liters a minute. Fifteen minutes after, he returned and my saturation with the nasal cannula on was 97 percent. He said that was excellent. He took the nasal cannula off and left. I don't know where he was trained, but a postoperative patient needs a little more than 88 percent of oxygen saturation to generate a paO_2 of 60. I couldn't believe that he took the nasal cannula away.

Then the time came for me to walk in the unit for the first time. The nurse and two nursing assistants were present. The nurse helped me stand while the nursing assistant said, "No, no, lay back." I returned to the bed, and the nursing assistant took my blood pressure; it was 100/62. She said that it was good and that I could get off the bed. This was indeed a joke because what she needed to do was tilts, an incomplete acronym for tilt table test—blood pressure laying flat, standing for two minutes, and taking the blood pressure again. A difference of more than ten points by diastolic suggests hypovolemia due to dehydration or bleeding. A difference of ten beats in the heart rate also is indicative of the same. That means that the patient should not walk or if stable, not walk alone. If any nausea or fainting exists, it may point to a vaso-vagal response to position change. It's a very common test in the ICU. I didn't say anything to embarrass anyone. I walked to the desk but felt very weak, even though I didn't say it. I would like to compliment a black female nurse who took excellent care of me. One evening as she was leaving, I said that I didn't need the Toradol, but she insisted. I know now that if she had left without giving me any, I would have had to wait a very long time for it.

I was discharged home the next day. I drove my van home. My wife and I went to Las Vegas the following Monday; I drove throughout the journey. I never went to a specific rehab but implemented my own. I never visited the ER for chest pain since that operation, but in April 10, 2012, it will be seventeen years post-op, and these grafts do not remain open for eternity.

After staying away from work for twenty-eight days, I was determined to return. I worked four hours every day for five days and then returned to my usual schedule of twelve-hour days. The ICUs were under renovation, to be combined into one large ICU. I don't know whose brainchild this was, but it was rejected by everyone. I was not against taking care of cardiac or medical patients, but a problem that arose if you were saddled with a medical and a surgical patient was that it may complicate your routine, especially if surgery doctors were going to insert a Swan and medical doctors were going to intubate someone. However, solving that problem rested with the charge nurse, the head nurse, and management. During the renovation of the ICU, we nurses were often providing care in some very unsafe situations, especially with intubated patients.

If I had to do this whole exercise over again, I might not change much—except, perhaps, that I needed at least three months off before returning to work, and I should have attended cardiac rehab. I thank God for bearing with me, for forgiving sins that are not easily absolved, and for giving me the time back to see my daughter grow and become independent. I thank all the cardiac surgeons that took care of me, and even those nurses that I thought needed retraining. My wife resigned from the MICU because she asked for emergency leave to take care of me and it was denied, so she left. She found two very good jobs in a month.

I have to say that after that cardiac surgery, I was a very angry man. I was so angry that I felt that I could shoot someone if they got in my way. I couldn't find the reason as to why I was so angry. I was angry at the army's doctors, who should have treated my cholesterol more aggressively; I was angry at them for not ordering a cardiac catheterization; and I was angry with myself for not guiding or insisting on better treatment. I had severe road rage if anyone had cut in front of me. There is a joke, which I usually tell my peers, that if you go to the army ER for a cut on your finger, you'll get a rectal examination. Of all the countries that I have visited and lived in, the United States doctors have a fetish for the priority they put on rectal examinations.

This anger that engulfed me took many, many years to subside, and often times when I am confronted with people with limited reasoning—especially those who are in clerical positions who treat errors as the norm because they can erase them and correct them—I really blow up. I cannot make those errors or I'd kill my patients, so I expect others to be a little more attentive and *pay attention to detail.* There was an entry in my cardiac operation records about air in the mechanical pump, and I think that the gap that exists between placing and replacing patients on the pump causes minor brain damage. This is my opinion and belief. I have also spoken with several open heart patients and they relate also to unprovoked anger. I now refer to it as the post-op disease process. It's not one that I could have controlled easily.

I thank my wife for entertaining my anger and guiding me back to civility after one of these angry episodes. I have prayed to God to guide and help me through this punishing era. This anger lasted almost ten years before subsiding to a 2/10 on a scale of 1-10. If others had known how angry I was, especially at inefficiency, they would have stayed very far away from me. Presently, I am more reserved and mellow. I accept the things that I cannot change but I still occasionally get angry when professionals try to bluff me and I know that they are incompetent. I quickly let them know that I am aware of their inefficiency.

I have made a study of fifty cardiac patients who have had cardiac operations (open heart), and 90 percent have told me that they experience the same anger. Then I further investigated cardiac patients with chest pain, those who have received stents, and I found that they also exhibit unexplained anger. This definitely gave me the advantage in taking care of cardiac patients. After a fifteen-minute chat with an angry patient, I usually am able to befriend them and remove much of the anger for I am one of them. I have experienced and can emit the empathy they deserve.

DESMOND S.

May I also say that stress is real. Previously, if anyone had said that they were stressed out, I'd tell them that I'd stress their ass out; but I have experienced stress. Sometimes it's not a phenomenon that can be explained, but you feel so fatigued, sometimes incoherent, and it's not something that you can easily turn on or off. I always try to relax when I feel this condition approaching.

THE MISTAKES THAT I HAVE MADE

I have looked at and described others' mistakes; let's look at mine. I was in Germany, and quite a lot of reservists were reporting for duty. Quite a few of them claimed that they had ICU experience, but you can work with a nurse for one hour and comfortably perceive whether they have had ICU experience or not. Perhaps they had ICU step-down experience. Good ICU nurses are a special breed of nurses. They are dedicated, vigilant commanders and rise to the occasion of excellence when needed. They advise doctors, correct doctors, assist in the training of interns and residents, and most of all, are patient advocates.

I was taking care of a brittle diabetic patient as an LVN, followed by a newly (to our ICU) registered reservist nurse. The doctor called and asked for the nurse that was taking care of the diabetic patient; the reservist ran to the phone and intimated that it was she. The doctor verbally gave the nurse orders to stop the five percent Dextrose solution and hang normal saline instead. She did not convey this to me, and it was caught by the following shift. This, of course, was chalked up as my mistake. As I intimated previously, I hate to make a mistake. The patient was not in any immediate danger, but the nurse said that she informed me. I was exceedingly skeptical working with the new reservist nurses again.

Some years later, I was orienting an aspiring LVN and I checked everything that he did very thoroughly. I really thought that I did so much with him that he was "shining." The last day, the last hour, the last drug was to be given thirty minutes before my shift ended. The patient had to have Pepcid (famotidine) by piggyback IV. I allowed him to get the med and hang it. He hung the right drug, the right amount, on the right patient, but with another patient's name written on the bag. It was in my patient's bin. I could have screwed his head off. It was discovered by the following shift. But that patient had left the ICU 3 days ago and the drug should have been received by pharmacy representatives.

So while orienting personnel in the ICU or any ward, don't ever let your guard down. Be vigilant and diligent, regardless of how clever and attentive your orientee is. I have learned from my mistakes, and those two errors never emerged again. But even more importantly, I've learned from other nurses' mistakes; I hope you will do the same. I have worked at a hospital ICU where a new, inexperienced nurse pushed 20 milliequivalants (meq) of potassium into a patient's veins. She had meant to introduce Lasix. Those were the days when nurses mixed their own potassium IV drug. However, coming to this nurse's defense, the unit stock of Lasix and potassium were in similar vials and situated side by side on the shelf. The patient showed no signs of any cardiac problems, but potassium is the drug of choice for condemned inmates' execution.

Whatever Happened in the OR?

Last but not least, this is the case of a patient who was going to have an operation referred to as UPPP (short for uvuloplatopharyngoplasty). The patient was later brought out with a tracheostomy, and the reason given was that the patient had coughed, lost his endotracheal tube, and the reintubation was extremely difficult and unsuccessful. Obviously, not enough oxygen was getting to his brain, and ultimately, he was pronounced brain dead. His brain stem reacted to suctioning and pain on arrival, but eventually faded and he was finally made a DNR (do not resuscitate). He subsequently passed. I felt especially for this guy and his wife, who did not understand the ultimate diagnosis.

This was a terrible accident, but I always wondered how anesthetists and anesthesiologists were comfortable bringing a patient from the OR with the ETT half secured. I was always terrified and ensured that an endotracheal tube holder was quickly put in place. I always wondered what the doctor told this patient's family. This incident was kept hushed up and not very many nurses spoke of it. I think that this was exclusive incompetence, malpractice, and an utter disregard for life.

A similar incident occurred when my patient was going to have a tracheostomy because of the inability to extubate an endotracheal tube. The longer the patient has an endotracheal tube, the more susceptible they are to acquiring infections, especially to the lungs.

What Went Wrong with an Intended Tracheostomy

The patient was briefed by the doctor and I; all papers were signed, and the patient was told of the right to refuse. I assured the patient that this procedure was often done at the bedside, in the ICU. I assured her that I would be present during the operation and everything would be okay. I now regret saying this because everything did not go okay.

We could not get anesthesia personnel's support—this is almost a red flag in the ICU—but I was also capable of administering medication and "bagging" the patient with 100 percent oxygen. The endotracheal tube of the patient was very small, and I heard the staff doctor say that there was some resistance going down the tube. The further he went, the more mucus blocked the sight of the laryngoscope. The staff doctor said that he could see where the resident was pushing on the trachea with a needle but could not see the needle, eventhough I saw the needle puncturing the skin above the 'Adam's apple'. This, I think, should have been the biggest red flag suggesting to everyone that this procedure should have been terminated until the staff could get a smaller laryngoscope, and even perform it in the operating room, with full anesthesia support.

The resident made about twenty punctures on the trachea, and finally, the blood pressure started to drop very quickly. Immediately the heart rate went into ventricular fibrillation, and the procedure changed into an open tracheotomy. CPR was done; every intervention failed. The patient's vital signs were stabilized, but the patient did not get adequate oxygen to the brain, which is the only explanation I can submit. The open incision was too long, and regardless of how much 100 percent oxygen was bagged into the lungs, the oximeter readings and blood gases were poor. I could have almost cried because I felt that I failed this patient miserably. Should I have insisted on having anesthesia personnel? Would that have made a difference? Should we have had more room to work?

These are questions that have rested with me for years, and I still cannot say for sure what the outcome would have been. Should they have done this procedure in the OR because of the small endotracheal tube? I think so, but I still don't know if it would have changed the results. I often wonder what the doctors told the family. I still feel that guilt and remorse.

Who Is the Teacher ?

I was specially selected to assist with a cardioversion. I could barely get a 20-gauge IV in the patient's right hand. The patient was a diabetic, in the seventies age group, and a very prominent figure in the community. The anesthetist was at the head of the bed, I was on the right and the cardiologist was on the left. This was a routine procedure because everyone knew exactly what their role would be. The cardiologist explained to the intern what the procedure was, what buttons to push on the defibrillator, and what rhythm to expect. The patient was counseled by myself and the cardiologist. The patient was admitted for a routine cardioversion of atrial fibrillation to sinus rhythm. The EKG monitor showed the patient's rhythm every second continuously. I sedated the patient, and he fell asleep.

The button was pushed after the desired current of fifty joules was selected. The monitor showed the impact, but the atrial fibrilation continued. The cardiologist intimated that the electricity needed to be raised. The intern raised the current to a hundred joules and, after sounding off "all clear," delivered the shock. I say shock because the intern did not push the sync button that changes the defibrillator from shocking mode to cardioversion. The patient's rhythm went into ventricular fibrillation when the intern had neglected to push the sync button.

The cardiologist quickly switched to two hundred joules, sounded all clear, and shocked the patient. There was a quiet calm in the patient's room because we were professionals except for one idiot. We started CPR as the rhythm did not change. The patient was shocked two more times before achieving sinus rhythm, but the blood pressure dropped and there was only the small 20-gauge IV. We needed to push fluids and start dopamine. Dopamine, a vasopressor or cardiac stimulant should only be infused through a central line into a large vein. Only doctors start these special lines on patients.

I received help from other nurses who were observing in getting an arterial line and a cordis prepared; someone called for a ventilator. The cordis and a-line were started, and dopamine was started. This immediately raised the blood pressure to an acceptable range. Blood gas and other laboratory blood were drawn and sent to the lab. The patient was medically stable but was placed on a ventilator for mechanical support. The patient was extubated that night but was kept in ICU and sent to the medical ward the next day. The patient was ultimately discharged in sinus rhythm, and he still had his life.

Lessons to Be Learned

- The patient came in for a routine procedure but ended up almost losing his life.
- There should have been more supervision on the intern. Never assume that they, interns, know.
- The patient was expected to leave the same day, but this incident hospitalized him for two days. The cost, obviously, was increased, and obviously this caused stress.
- The patient ended up not only with an IV but an NG (nasogastric) tube, an arterial line, a cordis, but with a ventilator as well. (Can you imagine how terrified the patient was after awakening?)
- The family had to be told the truth, as well as the patient after he/she became coherent.

Could this incident have been avoided? I will let you be the judge.

After that display, I have always added my own instruction to doctors and interns. I taught ACLS, so I was qualified to teach this subject. I always keep my eyes on the defibrillator and the buttons that operators used. To this one incident I say, "Thank God."

Last but Not Least

I have been given permission by my wife to write about some of her experiences. She was getting ready to pace a patient via a defibrillator and had the pacing pads in her hands when a fool turned the defibrillator on. My wife was shocked and had to be taken to the ER. No apologies can erase the pain and suffering of this error or, furthermore, the possibility of death.

My wife, who is also an intensive care nurse, was working on a ward in a hospital. We had just returned from Germany. The patient that a nurse was taking care of had a nasogastric tube, but Dietary had sent a full diet for the patient. The nurse came to my wife and said, "I can't get the beef down the tube. It only goes so far." She was stuffing beef and rice down the nasogastric tube. The doctor had failed to change the dietary order, but she should have informed the doctor of the error and have the diet changed to liquid.

There were also rumors while I was an LVN that a patient from a different hospital was given Mylanta (aluminum hydroxide), similar to Maalox, an antacid, via IV infusion. Mylanta is taken by mouth or down a nasogastric tube. I never knew how true this was, but after reading some of my examples, doubt is shaded with suspicion.

The last but not least example that I can relate is when, as charge nurse, I was working night shift, often referred to the graveyard shift. Quite a few nurses would not turn on the light in the patient's room when hanging medications. One nurse asked me to watch her patient as she was going to lunch. I accepted the task as it was part of my duty to ensure that all nurses ate while I covered their patients.

I entered the room after about ten minutes to ensure that the patient was okay and discovered that there was a maintenance IV running, a piggyback of antibiotics running at 5 cc/hr, and an insulin drip being given as a bolus. I immediately stopped the insulin drip, performed a blood sugar check, and found that the results were 27. The patient was a diabetic. I immediately pushed one amp of dextrose. I rechecked the glucose, and it was 117. I informed the doctor and requested a post-administration order.

I am a diabetic, and if my glucose goes below 60, my eyes become blurred, so I am very much aware not only by the literature but personal experience too. I reprimanded the nurse and wrote a complaint. If I did not visit this patient's room, he could have died from hypoglycemia. I have family who died from hypoglycemia.

Violence in the Workplace

There was an incident that occurred in the ICU where the charge nurse ordered a solid, hardcore elder and experienced nurse to clean a particular room. Unpleasant words were exchanged, for the nurse expressed the view that the room had been empty for hours and the charge nurse could have gotten off the buttocks and cleaned/prepared it. However, the nurse went to the room and started cleaning it. The charge nurse left the break room and went to the room, stood at the door, and imitated a chicken by clucking and waving his elbows up and down. This was a little disrespectful to the nurse, so he chased the charge nurse around the unit and punched the nurse; it was a trap. The charge nurse called for help and shouted for security to be called. Statements were gathered, the nurse was forced to resign, and the charge nurse was reported to the licensing board. How stupid, but it happens.

There were at least two incidents involving me. The first was in the SICU, an open-bay ICU, and I had two post-op patients on ventilators. The surgeon made a change on the ventilator but did not record it on the respiratory tech's flow sheet, so he turned the ventilator settings back to its original. He was still there when I looked at the ventilator and saw that the setting was incorrect. I confronted the respiratory tech and inquired if he did that; his reply was that the doctor had not written the order. It was usual for the surgeons to change the settings of the ventilator and leave it for twenty minutes, order a blood gas, and make further changes or assessments. This really angered me for regardless if the surgeon was right or not, the patient's life was in the middle.

I told him that I was right there between the two beds, and if he had brought it to my attention, I would have written the order for the doctor; the doctor would then have co-signed it later. The doctor was in the OR. I took his file of orders and discovered that he (the tech) did not even have an order sheet prepared. I threw this file about four beds away. The next day, the technician's supervisor approached me to rebuke my actions, but I felt so disgusted with the technician's actions that I refused to listen to what he had to say. I think the supervisor reported me to my head nurse. I was never told what came out of the matter. That technician was forced to resign or fired about six months after this incident. Some document was entered into my file, but I was never admonished.

I intimated earlier how difficult taking care of two critically ill patients could be. This is a very good example, but it is also an example of an incompetent charge nurse. I can talk about this incident because I personally was involved. I had a postoperative (surgical) and a medical patient. At 4 a.m. I drew blood on both. The postoperative patient had a Swan-Ganz but no arterial line. Obviously, he had no arterial line because he was a difficult stick, but a blood gas was ordered. After at least two attempts, I got the arterial blood gas from the radial artery. The medical patient also had a blood gas ordered—no arterial line. I stuck him and got the blood gas with other ordered labs.

Another nurse came over to help me and started labeling the blood. The nurse labeled them incorrectly while the charge nurse, who initially was a cardiac nurse, looked on. I rushed the blood down to the lab. I was called fifteen minutes later, and the tech told me that there was a mislabeling of the blood. I replied that I was not sure what else could be done, but I knew that I had to redraw the blood. He called me twice again, and all he had to do was discard the blood. By this time, the medical patient started to vomit blood. I had to introduce a nasogastric tube and lavage with normal saline. This calling on the phone really irritated me as I had to work on this bleeding patient very quickly to prevent hypovolemia. I said, "Don't call me again" and "f—k you." This obviously was because of the frustration from inadequate help from the charge nurse, who was in the sixties age group, but also with the mislabeling of the blood by another nurse.

The tech showed up at my ICU threatening to "kick my ass." He was my friend, but I was not going to back down. If at any time anyone punches me or attempts to punch me, he'll get it. The size of opponents never scared me. After about five minutes of exchanging of words, which the charge nurse seemed to enjoy, the tech left. That tech and I have worked together again several times, but our friendship was ruined. We only exchanged information on patients and said hi when we passed.

Then the investigation and trial began. The team consisted of the chief nurse, the head nurse, and the assistant head nurse. I was not scared or intimidated by this inquiry. Before they started their admonishment—and because I knew I was wrong—I admitted that I was wrong, that I was the professional, and that it should never have occurred and never will again. But I also vented my disgust on the charge nurse for not intervening to help with my patients and standing idly by. After I spoke, there was no more that anyone could say that would elevate the unfortunate incident. The head nurse repeated what I had said, and the matter was considered closed. I honestly regret this incident to this day. I know that I have more tolerance, integrity and discipline than I displayed.

With this last example of unfortunate incidents, I hope that whoever reads these will not repeat them.

I was not present but there was no doubt in my mind that the following is true. There was a cardiologist who threw instruments indiscreetly, sometimes hitting his staff. He is a very excellent cardiologist, but was sometimes weird.

He often spoke on one subject and would jump to another, similar to a flight of ideas. He was transferred, ultimately.

What a Nurse Needs to Know to Perform

Lesson 1 is to know your limits. Never be ashamed to say, "I don't know, but I will find out." You are part of an intricate network called a team. The team will support you, but the team is only as strong as the weakest link. Competition between teams is healthy, meaning that whichever team shows more cohesion and adhesion, gets more recognition. Doctors, nurses and patients like efficient, proficient, knowledgeable and skillful teams. Teams also assist each other, and if that doesn't exist, then the charge nurse / head nurse should intervene.

There is no such thing as a "best" nurse because standards across the nation and the states vary significantly, so the question that should be asked is, what measuring tool should be used to assess performance? Some hospitals' policies provides for nurses to pull chest tubes, while others don't. So this one example proves the point of capability. A nurse is only strong and efficient because of the cooperation, knowledge, and dedication of peers. No nurse should say that they are the best in the unit as this can only be judged by peers and patients. Humility is a virtue in health care, and should be practiced on entry to the profession. Have you ever thought that regardless of how good you are, there is always someone better the world over? The heading of this paragraph should end with *efficiently*. You must know all the patients on the unit, their diagnoses, and their status: DNR (do not resuscitate), full code, do not intubate but can have electricity, etc. Do not perform CPR on a DNR patient. Read your hospital and unit policies; read and understand HIPPA regulations. The latter discussion includes patient privacy laws. Ensure you get enough sleep and rest or you can't perform efficiently.

Dedication

If you are in the nursing profession for money and a job, you are surely in the wrong profession. Dedication in nursing is intertwined with devotion, pledging, and instrumentally becoming a patient advocate. A nurse has to be honest, knowledgeable, wholehearted, selfless, empathic, and tender to all patients, doctors, and peers. There is not one aspect of dedication that can be ignored; all principles must be observed. Love your expertise, your profession, your patients, and your peers. This type of true dedication cannot be achieved in a year but graduates as time progresses. Dedication involves knowledge. I read on the Internet a little list of inspiration/motivation published by Tully NewsInfo:

10 Ways to Love.

1. Listen without interrupting. (Proverbs 18).
2. Speak without accusing. (James 1:19).
3. Give without sparing. (Proverbs 21:26).
4. Pray without ceasing. (Colossians 1:9).
5. Answer without arguing. (Proverbs 17:1).
6. Share without pretending. (Ephesians 4:15).
7. Enjoy without complaint. (Philippics 4:15).
8. Trust without wavering. (Corinthians 13:7).
9. Forgive without punishing. (Colossians).
10. Promise without forgetting. (Proverbs 13:12).

Forget the scripture entry; the mere meaning of these words can motivate many.

Qualification

Know your limits; I cannot stress this enough, especially to new nurses to this field. Know when to call the doctor and call for help. You'd be surprised how many other nurses, your peers, know and can help immediately. Remember that nursing is team effort. We always depend on each other.

Obviously, it's excellent to be qualified, but being qualified, knowledgeable, skillful, and wise are separate entities of qualification. There are some who are perpetual students, obtaining a master's in nursing without having any or very little experience, especially in the ICU. There are so many new equipment and procedures arriving yearly or monthly, and changes in policy happen almost inadvertently. The basics often remain the same, but it would be wise to get some experience as your qualification improves. I can almost name two to three nurses that have master's degrees who never did perform very well in the ICU. There were several that came as head nurses with master's degrees that couldn't admit a patient quickly and efficiently. Some went through multiple episodes of orientation and still had to be removed from the ICU. By the same token, I can name a few with whom I was very impressed. Attending college and gaining knowledge are not synonymous.

They should be, but there are some who do the mere minimum to graduate and there are those who graduate and quickly forget the principles of nursing. And there are the very lazy ones and the complainers. One does not have to attend college to possess knowledge, but the "proof of the pudding" is in the eating. So skills are developed through practice, trial and error; and wisdom is achieved by the application of knowledge. Wisdom is not accomplished in months but in years, and it's a virtue, almost immaculate. I am certain that there are many times you wonder, *Where did this nurse train or graduate?* This is the exception to the rule of nurturing the new nurse, training and educating the new graduate. New nurses are always welcome—the more, the merrier—but they must demonstrate that desire to learn.

There are a lot of books written on nursing, and quite a few are written as a thesis for a master's program. But the authors of many that I have read seem to have been lost in oblivion in trying to develop and create new phrases and titles, as if they were developing something completely new. There are some that I've read that fail to qualify and quantify nursing. Yet there is a very prominent university that accepts that kind of literature for students. So my view is that qualification does not necessarily produce a good nurse. Likewise, I have seen a few doctors pass through the cracks, unfortunately. Some were placed on probation and still could not start an arterial line or insert a cordis. It's unbelievable, but they passed.

Areas of Nursing

Usually, after a year or so, a nurse may be able to decide which branch of nursing suits them the most. I would like to vehemently document that ICU nursing cannot be accomplished from the nurse's desk. You should have the patient and the monitor in your view most of the time. So if a nurse has chosen the ICU, it's consistently hard, complicated work. But those who are involved in noncontact patient care should have the knowledge and skills to perform in any department.

Make it your duty to know about other departments, units, and wards. A rule of thumb is to give in-services. I've always contended that if you can teach a subject, you know the subject—that is, if it was well-prepared and well-delivered. So you do not have to be the "education" nurse to teach, just do not overstretch the topic in length and time, but prepare well. Prepare answers to questions that you may be asked, so that you can answer without hesitation. There is usually one person in an audience or group that you are teaching who will ask that question that you did not perceive.

Look and Learn

A very valuable tool is to look and learn. If you don't know, say that you don't know; peers will respect you for your honesty. Know your limitations and don't guess. I have learned a lot by observing, asking, finding out, and finally, applying. I am what I am because of the help of my peers.

Defensive Charting

There are some hospitals that have flow sheets where you can mark off *what*, *where*, and *when*. But you need to address at least two problems of the patient. I have always used the SOAPIER method of charting. You will need to say in what state the patient was at the beginning of your shift and address the progression or regression at the end of your shift.. If the patient's condition deteriorated at the end of your shift, document so. It's not necessarily your fault. For instance, if the patient is being treated for an infection and is receiving antibiotics, not unless the immune system kicks in will the infection subside.

S—subjective. Even though the patient only says "good morning," this shows orientation, and it's an asset in the ICU where some patients are drugged up, don't see the sun, and the atmosphere sounds like an episode from Star Wars, especially at night. The alarms are usually set to detect abnormality, but not in every case will there be an intervention. You can learn a lot from verbal interaction with the patient. Encourage conversation but know when to quit.

O—your observation. Look, listen, feel. Do you here crackles, rales, heart murmurs, bowel sounds? Are they active, hypoactive, or hyperactive? Is there any distention? When was the last bowel movement, and are you concerned about the time? Report your abnormal findings to the doctor. Do any of their lab values stick out? Generally speaking, how do they look? Are they in pain? Look at their pupils, you can assess a lot from them.

A—your assessment. In the ICU you are allowed to use broad terms, such as hemodynamic stability, alteration in, related to, hypotension, grade 4 murmur, bradycardia with multifocal PVCs, Hx of CABG in 1995, grade 2 pitting edema in lower extremities, febrile at 38 degrees, respiratory dysfunction related to vent dependency, rales throughout bases of lungs, febrile, pneumonia, and so on.

P—your plan for this patient for the day, such as giving Tylenol as ordered; initiating incentive sphirometer if the patient is alert and not on a ventilator; lowering room temperature; reporting murmurs, edema, and temperature to attending physician; suctioning patient as required and prn; documenting the color, consistency, and amount of sputum; weaning patient off the ventilator, and so on.

I—your interventions: suctioned for large, dark brown, thick secretions from lungs; MD notified and specimen sent to lab; MD notified of all findings and plan carried out; applied elastic stockings or PAS to lower extremities; bed bath was done; patient should be kept clean and tidy at all times; and so on. Whatever you do should be documented. If you didn't get to something because of more important procedures, document it and pass it on to the next shift.

E—evaluate if the suctioning helped the crackles, describe the fever. Is it still there or is it subsiding? Are the stockings decreasing the edema? Stockings (and also PAS) should be taken off once a shift, every shift, for at least one hour. Did the antipyretic and bath help the fever? And so on.

R—reevaluation: are the interventions helping the patient? Are there any more doctor's orders? What is the significant improvement? And so on.

I have used similar notes, and the Joint Commission team that looked at my patient and notes were very impressed that I was addressing the patient's problems and also with the manner of my presentation.

So this is a crude example, but you should get the idea. Never chart anything that you didn't do; pass the task on to the following shift and say why it was not accomplished. A trauma patient may have arrived, another patient may have "crashed," and so on.

The most important aspect of nursing is planning your work and working your plan. Help your peers; even if they did not ask for help, volunteer to help. This builds a good rapport with your peers. Compliment your peers for their good work, which brings us to the topic of supervision.

THE ONE MINUTE MANAGER

There are three basic rules of the "one minute manager." I have seen at least five nurses apply these principles. I am going to be as concise and precise as possible. These three rules, regardless of their brevity, are worth a pot of gold in supervising.

1. On-the-spot correction: if you see something wrong, present it to the nurse. You should not only point out what is wrong, but add that you know that the nurse is a good person and that the correction is not personal, but it's the performance that needs reviewing. If possible, teach them how. If you wait to tell them a month away at their evaluation, they may even forget that any such thing occurred.

2. Walk around the unit early in the morning, and ask the staff how they are doing. Compliment them on their good work. I remember when chief nurses walked around the unit and chatted with us for about two minutes or so. On other times, as chief nurses change, I often wondered who was the chief nurse because I never saw them. By visiting a unit, you will create a bond with your nurses, and when the head nurse speaks about them, the chief nurse will know who they are. They will have a picture in their mind of whom the head nurse is speaking.

3. Especially the head nurse, it is expected that an early morning visit should be made so as to greet the night shift and the day shift. Hold short meetings to discuss problems, and if you can't answer immediately, say you will find out, and do so. Set the tone and culture of the unit. This applies to chief nurses, head nurses, unit supervisors, and charge nurses.

4.   Reward good performance. Let the nurse know that you are aware of the good work performed. If possible, a reward can come later, but the praise should be immediate. The ICU that I worked in had a very unusual, dynamic head nurse in that she was able to motivate over twenty-five nurses to challenge the CCRN examination and pass. She was one of the very few head nurses that were knowledgeable, could take care of critical patients, and was an asset in a code blue function. I was sorry when she left because we got stuck with one who was more interested in rank and status than motivating, structuring, and inviting cohesion and adhesion to the unit.

5.   This is the first time that I have used gender, but she deserves the praise. There would always be "criers" in the unit, but the majority of staff appreciated what she accomplished. I take my hat off to such tact and excellence. She also displayed a high regard for ethics. The greatest asset of ethical behavior is honesty, and you can bet that if there was something wrong, you'd surely hear about it. She undoubtedly possessed that great charm that allowed you to feel appreciated. I am sure that she'll excel in any branch of nursing that she accepts. On behalf of our ICU unit, I extend our greatest thank you to this head nurse. She was our greatest asset.

Laboratory Values and Their Meanings

I am not going to elaborate on this subject, but it is necessary that the nurse is knowledgeable of laboratory values since, most times, the nurse gets them before the doctor. The nurse should be able to assess these values as normal or abnormal, especially the standard values of a renal panel, a metabolic panel, liver enzymes, cardiac enzymes, a CBC (complete blood count), Pt/PTT (prothrombin time/partial prothrombin time), and the other minute values of drugs such as vancomycin, digoxin, TSH level, etc. This knowledge and practice can save many a life. There may be standing orders that give you the privilege of drawing blood if the nurse sees any abnormalities such as dysrrhythmias/arrhythymias as these may point to electrolyte imbalance, especially in potassium and magnesium. Decreased sodium is more connected to disorientation. From a renal panel, you can assess kidney function, which is particularly valuable if the patient will have a CT with contrast. Metabolic panels can detect liver function from ALT (alanine aminotransferase), AST (aspartate aminotransferase serum), and GGT (gamma-glutamyl transpeptidase). A CBC can tell you about anemia or possible bleeding or infection and your platelet count. Amylase and lipase tests are very important. Some laboratories do not run lipase unless it is specifically ordered.

When giving medications by IV, they should be placed in a pump unless you are giving a bolus through a very fragile vein. So you should make yourself aware of the functions of a pump. Most pumps can calculate and deliver medications by calculating micrograms per kilogram per minute. Some medications—I am certain you are familiar with are dopamine and dobutamine—are always infused as micrograms per kilogram per minute. If the dose readings give 10 mcg/kg/min, the weight of the patient is 165 lb and the concentration of the medication is 500 mg in 250 cc. You must be able to calculate this so as to ensure that the pump is correct.

I am not going to irritate you with calculations, but you really need to know them, especially if they were started without a pump being installed immediately for some legitimate reason, such as being in the heart catheterization lab and have to calculate micrograms per cc/ml. Medications make the patient comfortable during procedures, and always give reassurance, hope, and comfort. This brings the rest of this book to patients' rights and responsibilities.

Patients' Rights and Responsibilities

When you are in the hospital, you are a customer. You are receiving services that you are paying to be given. You have the right to excellent health care in any hospital. Don't ever be afraid to ask questions; you are not only entitled to, but expected to ask.

THE OTHER SIDE OF THE MEDICAL COIN

You have the right to know the name of the hospital, the ward/unit on which floor you're on, and the names of your doctors and nurses.

You have the right to

1. know your diagnosis;
2. know the health care team's plan;
3. know what medications you are receiving and why;
4. know the side effects of the medication and the specific reaction and how it will react with other drugs you are taking (compatibility);
5. ask about hand washing from doctors, nurses, and visitors;
6. ask about checking your ID (usually on your hand) from all staff before any procedures, especially from those giving medication;
7. ask about any tests that you are informed that they will perform. Ask at what time they will be performed, why are they needed, how they will be performed, and when the results will be ready;
8. ask the nurse how long you may be hospitalized and what their plan for discharge is;
9. take notes or have a friend or relative write down relevant points of your illness and care;
10. be oriented to the unit/ward. Keep the call bell in reach. Do not get out of bed alone and wait for health care personnel's presence/help. You may have sedatives in your system that may make you dizzy on standing. You may be dehydrated and become dizzy when you stand;
11. ask for any literature on your illness;
12. be entitled to the results of your tests and a copy of your records;
13. call for help if needed;
14. report any unusual feelings;
15. have visiting time included in your orientation;
16. be in charge. You have the right to refuse any treatment, but with refusal occasionally comes medical consequences;
17. have the right to know about your progress;

18. have the right to know if the treatment is experimental and if it is necessary for you to give written permission;
19. have the right to express your spiritual and cultural values, provided they do not annoy or interrupt medical treatment;
20. be advised about the need for a power of attorney or to appoint a surrogate to make decisions for you if the need arises;
21. receive adequate and prompt responses to your questions;
22. know the rules and regulations of the hospital;
23. have the right to medical care regardless of your race, sex, creed, sexual orientation, national origin, religion, or even sources of payment;
24. have the right to privacy relatively;
25. have the right to complain if not satisfied with your care; and
26. have your health care record shared only with those on a "need-to-know basis."

Your Responsibilities

You need to know the responsibilities of refusing treatment:

- Understand the plan of care.
- If your condition changes, report it to the nurse immediately.
- Be polite to hospital staff and be considerate of the rights of other patients.
- Report the most accurate and complete information on your medical condition—both past and present—and any drugs you have taken, prescribed or over the counter.
- Cover your mouth when coughing; get rid of all used napkins.
- Prepare your advanced directives, including directives to physicians, surrogate bodies, and family. This should be signed, witnessed, dated, notarized, and placed in your medical record. You should not be compelled by anyone to make this document, but it helps to direct your care if you are unable to write or speak.

- Report pain, including onset; the anatomical position of pain-point to area; if it's present all the time or intermittent; and what makes it worse or better. On a scale of 1—10, how would you rate the pain, with 1 being the lowest and 10 the highest in intensity? If you are medicated, how much pain remains and for how long?

- Provide your insurance card/cards. You are responsible for the deductible as determined by your insurance. If you are covered by more than one insurance plan, usually the latter pays the deductible. More than often, you have to direct the hospital on how to bill both insurance companies.

- On discharge, you should know the time so you can call a relative/ friend and check your bathroom for glasses or teeth (if you have false teeth); your purse, and any of your money/documents stored in the hospital safe. Ensure that you know what medications you will be taking, their purposes, and their side effects.

Good luck to all.

Special thanks to

Those responsible for my orientation and education,

Martha	Ronnie	Rose	Liz	Carol

Maria	Elizabeth	Mary	Christine	Christine

Those I owe for their dedicated cooperation,

Susan	Pat	Beth	Jimenez	Abel	Rose	Jana

Jaime	Michael	Nancy	Nancy	Pamela	Gary	Betty

Harvey	Linda	All unit clerks

And those who inspired and motivated me.

Jana	Rose	Beth

And all ICU staff.

BIBLIOGRAPHY

Saunders Nursing Drug Handbook 2009, Appendix A

The American Century Thesaurus, published by the Oxford University Press, original edition.

"Ten Ways to Love" from http://www.facebook.com/chakriya.uv

The One Minute Manager, Kenneth Blanchard, Ph.D
Spencer Johnson, M.D.